CRANIOFACIAL ANOMALIES

A Beginner's Guide for Speech-Language Pathologists

CRANIOFACIAL ANOMALIES

A Beginner's Guide for Speech-Language Pathologists

ALICE KAHN, Ph.D.

Speech-Language Pathology
Department of Communication
Miami University
Oxford, Ohio

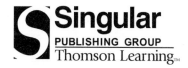

Singular
PUBLISHING GROUP
Thomson Learning™

Singular Publishing Group
Thomas Learning
401 West A Street, Suite 325
San Diego, California 92101-7904

Singular Publishing Group, Inc., publishes textbooks, clinical manuals, clinical reference books, journals, videos, and multimedia materials on speech-language pathology, audiology, otorhinolaryngology, special education, early childhood, aging, occupational therapy, physical therapy, rehabilitation, counseling, mental health, and voice. For your convenience, our entire catalog can be accessed on our web-site at **http//www.singpub.com**. Our mission to provide you with materials to meet the daily challenges of the ever changing health care/educational environment will remain on course if we are in touch with you. In that spirit, we welcome your feedback on our products. Please telephone (**1-800-521-8545**), fax (**1-800-774-8398**), or e-mail (**singpub@singpub.com**) your comments and requests to us.

© 2000 by Singular Publishing Group

Typeset in 10/12 Palatino by So Cal Graphics
Printed in the United States of America by West Group

Library of Congress Cataloging-in-Publication Data

Kahn, Alice, 1946–
    Craniofacial anomalies : a beginner's guide for speech-language pathologists / by Alice Kahn.
        p.   cm.
    Includes bibliographical references and index.
    ISBN 1-56593-987-5 (soft cover : alk. paper)
    1. Head—Abnormalities—Diagnosis.   2. Face—Abnormalities—Diagnosis.   3. Speech therapists.   I. Title.
    [DNLM: 1. Craniofacial Abnormalities—diagnosis.   WE 705 K12c 2000]
RD763K34   2000
617.5′1—dc21
DNLM/DLC
for Library of Congress   99-40682
                                                                    CIP

CONTENTS

PREFACE

As a speech pathologist teaching in a nonmedical university setting, I have often envied colleagues who are members of a craniofacial team. The opportunity to use "cutting edge" technology, participate in interdisciplinary planning in a medical environment, and observe long-term surgical results has always seemed an extraordinary professional asset.

Fortunately, those of us working in environments far removed from craniofacial teams can also have extraordinary professional opportunities if we know where and how to look for them. We can begin by remembering that undiagnosed patients with craniofacial anomalies are always present in our work settings and are sometimes already a part of our clinical caseloads. Although individuals with obvious craniofacial anomalies are usually diagnosed at birth, individuals with less apparent craniofacial anomalies may be misdiagnosed, undiagnosed, or simply unrecognized by health care professionals. Our problem is not lack of clinical opportunity, but lack of skill in recognizing and interpreting subtle indications of craniofacial involvement.

Speech-language pathology students often want to know why an understanding of embryology and craniofacial anatomy is necessary for someone who has no plans to work in a medical setting. The answer is simple: Patients with craniofacial anomalies are found in all clinical settings and not all have yet been accurately identified and treated. Some of the best clinicians I know are those who practice the art of clinical observation. These individuals have learned to how to make accurate diagnoses by relating their observations to an anatomical knowledge base and by then using their conclusions to develop and implement an appropriate plan of long-term patient care.

Clinical observation is an art, one that is similar to photography. I have often heard someone compliment a photographer by saying, "What a great photograph! You must have a really good camera." Few people realize that the "art" of photography depends not on an expensive camera, but on the ability of the photographer to observe a scene and to translate this image onto film. Clinical observation, like photographic observation, is a learned art that can be obtained with training and refined with practice.

The purpose of this book is to help you acquire or improve the observational techniques needed to assess patients who may have undiagnosed craniofacial anomalies. The information in this book can help you learn how to use anatomical information as a diagnostic tool. It will also help you learn how to observe, identify, and document the presence of minor birth anomalies in patients. Finally, you will learn how to interpret your observations, make referrals to appropriate professionals, and report your findings to patients and family members.

This book begins with an introduction to the art of observation and continues with Chapter 2, "Building a Knowledge Base: Concepts of Craniofacial Development." This chapter contains a basic review of anatomical information pertinent to craniofacial growth and development. Normal facial growth and development, as well as a comparison of normal racial differences in craniofacial structure, are discussed here.

Protocols for observing orofacial structures are described in Chapter 3, "Learning to Observe: Collecting Information." Sensitive issues and ethical considerations related to craniofacial assessment are also included.

Chapter 4, "Understanding Your Observations: Differential Diagnosis and Patient Disposition," addresses methods of interpreting diagnostic information and planning for patient treatment or referral. Material that will help you learn to distinguish between birth anomalies and those caused by accidents, medication, or disease processes are found in this chapter.

Chapter 5, "Writing Readable Clinical Materials," provides suggestions for preparing educational materials for functionally illiterate patients. The topic of functional illiteracy and its impact on development of clinical materials is addressed here.

Chapter 6, "Building a Professional Support System," describes ways of building a support system for you and for your patients. Information in this chapter features development of patient support groups and ethical use of the Internet.

Finally, Chapter 7, "Photodocumenting Your Observations," provides the basic information you will need to make accurate permanent records of visual observations. Because photo documentation requires written patient consent, the ethical aspects of visual record keeping are discussed in this chapter.

Although craniofacial observation is often the first step in a patient's treatment plan, it is seldom the last. Many patients receiving treatment at major craniofacial centers were referred to those centers by skilled observers practicing in nonmedical settings. Skilled and accurate observation is a crucial first step in the treatment of patients with subtle craniofacial anomalies. Subtly affected patients are at the greatest risk of being misdiagnosed or undiagnosed. Skilled observers are always alert for the unexpected, always ready to take a second look on the patient's behalf. Although comparatively few of us will become members of a craniofacial team, all of us can learn the skills necessary to recognize, diagnose, refer, and treat the patients with craniofacial anomalies we encounter in our own work settings.

ACKNOWLEDGMENTS

I wish to thank those persons who agreed to be photographed and used as illustrations in this textbook. I am especially grateful to Wang Kai, a Miami University graduate student, for assistance in recruiting individuals to serve as models of normal patient appearance.

I am also grateful for the financial assistance provided by individuals in the College of Arts and Science and the Department of Communication at Miami University in support this project.

My graduate assistant, Jill Brown, deserves credit and thanks for organizing and formatting material in the Appendix. I am also extremely grateful to graphic artist Sara Udstuen and other artists in Miami University's Department of Applied Technologies who did far more than they had to do toward producing professional, camera-ready tables and figures. I am especially grateful to Gail Johnson, who organized production of tables and figures, and whose consistently cheerful assistance continued from start to finish. Finally, I wish to thank my friends Dr. Kathy Hutchinson, Dr. Laura Kelly, Dr. Daria Mauer, and Dr. Mary Pannbacker for providing encouragement throughout the course of this project.

This book is dedicated to my Father and to Grant.

CHAPTER 1

INTRODUCTION: THE ART OF OBSERVATION

Clinical observation is a learned art that can be practiced in any setting. Although the words *seeing* and *observing* are sometimes used interchangeably, the two concepts have quite different meanings. *Seeing* requires only that you have adequate eyesight to view an object. *Observing* requires you to recognize, identify, and analyze what you have seen. As a clinical observer you need time, good vision, a knowledge base, and intelligence to reach accurate conclusions. You must also remain alert and interested in the task at hand.

All of us recall times when we have mistakenly driven past a freeway exit while traveling a familiar route on the highway. Although we *saw* the signs announcing the upcoming exit, we did not *observe* their significance. Events like these often happen during familiar, repetitious, or boring activities. Because observation requires an active thought process, we are more likely to observe challenging, stimulating or interesting situations.

Diagnostic screenings and initial therapy sessions usually retain our interest because they are professionally challenging. Theoretically, such settings provide ideal opportunities to practice the art of clinical observation and to incorporate observational findings into therapy recommendations. In practice, however, the visual observation portion of a diagnostic session is often confined to a cursory examination of the patient's oral peripheral mechanism. If previous diagnostic reports are available, even a cursory examination may be omitted. Students in particular are often reluctant to perform detailed craniofacial examinations or to question the results of previous diagnostic reports.

Speech pathologists are sometimes reluctant to make craniofacial observation a part of the diagnostic process simply because doing so would require reorganizing examination procedures or developing new examination or patient-consent forms. These issues are actually time management concerns and can be easily resolved if there is a genuine desire to incorporate craniofacial observation into the diagnostic process. Concerns resulting from mistaken beliefs about the diagnostic process, however, are not so easily overcome.

DIAGNOSTIC MISCONCEPTIONS

A Physician Has Already Observed This Patient's Craniofacial Anatomy (Therefore I Don't Need To)

One of the most prevalent diagnostic misconceptions is that if a medical doctor provides us with a patient's records, we have no need to conduct additional anatomical observations of that patient. When we receive a physician's referral, it is easy to assume that all the patient's anatomical problems have been accurately identified. Sometimes they have; often, they have not.

The idea that all physicians are highly trained clinical observers is pervasive, but not entirely accurate. Although the majority of physicians receive extensive diagnostic training during medical school, that training is not necessarily concentrated in diagnosis of craniofacial anomalies, genetic problems, or communication disorders. Because observers see what they are trained to see, their ability to accurately diagnose craniofacial anomalies depends largely on the amount of specialized clinical training they have received. Time and financial constraints prevent even the most rigorous medical programs from teaching physicians to diagnose every potential medical problem. Many physicians (and many speech-language pathologists) complete their training with little or no experience in recognizing craniofacial anomalies.

The Physician's Diagnosis Is Always Correct

Academic or medical titles are unquestionably impressive, sometimes more impressive than the human being who holds the title. In any case, medical doctors and Ph.D.s are human, and even with extensive training and impressive titles they can make diagnostic mistakes. Although clinicians understand that competent professionals can make mistakes, information contained in medical reports is generally accepted at face value—especially if the report originates from a highly respected member of the medical community. Diagnostic mistakes do occur, and professionals should interpret medical reports cautiously, using them as a starting point in the diagnostic process. Serious mistakes can occur when clinicians allow information contained in medical reports to substitute for observations that should be obtained during diagnostic evaluations. The following case study illustrates a situation in which speech pathologists accepted assumptions contained in medical reports, thereby contributing to the physicians' diagnostic mistakes:

Jacques, a 23-year-old man of French-Canadian descent, lived and attended public schools in Baton Rouge, Louisiana, until age 18. His pediatrician noted that Jacques' physical development was normal, his only major health problem being repeated bouts of otitis media during infancy. These were treated successfully with antibiotics and caused no lasting hearing impairment. When Jacques was 6 years old, his family moved across town, and he was seen by another pediatrician. This physician noted that Jacques' conversational speech was slightly hypernasal, but the hypernasality did not interfere with speech intelligibility. Because Jacques' first and preferred spoken language was French, the pediatrician attributed the hypernasal quality to his use of Cajun dialect while speaking English. After entering elementary school, Jacques received semi-annual public school speech and hearing screenings. The school speech pathologists also noticed the hypernasal quality of Jacques' speech, but agreed with the pediatricians' diagnosis and did not recommend in-depth evaluation or enrollment in speech therapy. After graduating from high school, Jacques received a physical examination from a U.S. Army physician prior to enlisting in the armed services. This physician performed an oral examination and observed the presence of a bifid uvula. He was unable to detect the presence of the posterior nasal spine of the hard palate upon palpation. Radiographic and

(continued)

endoscopic observation confirmed that Jacques had a submucous cleft palate and inconsistent and insufficient velopharyngeal closure during conversational speech. Surgical remediation to improve velopharyngeal closure and eliminate hypernasal resonance was performed, and at age 20, the young man was able to speak with normal resonance for the first time in his life.

The above example indicates the danger of *assuming* the cause of a condition, rather than *observing* the cause of it. This patient had been *seen* by two physicians who assumed that the patient's resonance problem was related to dialectical issues, and by several speech pathologists who accepted the physicians' assumptions as facts. Because none of the health care professionals carefully *observed* the structure and function of the patient's oral peripheral mechanism, 20 years passed before the patient received accurate diagnosis and treatment.

Once Is Enough

Mistakes can also occur when diagnostic observations are viewed as permanent and unchanging records of the patient's oral-facial structure and function. We, as speech pathologists, often reevaluate a patient hoping to see progress in language usage or phoneme acquisition. Although age-related changes in communication skills are expected, we sometimes forget that the patient's oral-facial structures also undergo constant growth and age-related changes. Anatomical alterations may also occur as a result of disease, trauma, or surgical procedures. Because such changes can occur quickly and produce lasting effects on communication skills, oral-facial examinations should become a routine part of the reevaluation process.

What if I Make a Mistake?

Diagnostic mistakes occur, ironically, when we neglect to do a craniofacial examination for fear of making a mistake. Fear of making mistakes usually results from ignorance on our part. We, like physicians, often begin our careers without the specialized skills needed to treat all possible communication disorders. Fortunately, fear of making mistakes can be overcome by learning the techniques of observation and by putting these techniques into routine practice. The information in this book will help you acquire the knowledge base and observational skills you will need to make accurate and informed diagnostic decisions. The diagnostic process is never risk free, but it is always exciting. May you have the courage to continue learning and to use what you learn to make positive changes in the lives of patients in your care.

CHAPTER 2

BUILDING A KNOWLEDGE BASE: CONCEPTS OF CRANIOFACIAL DEVELOPMENT

As we observe someone whose facial appearance differs from normal, we often assume that this abnormal appearance has a genetic basis. Although genetic errors account for a substantial portion of craniofacial anomalies, other factors can also affect craniofacial appearance. Craniofacial anomalies may be caused by deformation of the developing fetus, by in-utero teratogens, or by neoplasms. Other causes of unusual craniofacial appearance include the effects produced by trauma, burn, long-term illness, or radiation exposure. Sometimes craniofacial "anomalies" are not anomalies at all, but normal racial variation in facial appearance. Because differential diagnosis is a fundamental part of our task as health care professionals, we must be able to distinguish between etiologies and to recognize the difference between normal and abnormal craniofacial features. Our task becomes easier if we understand basic concepts of craniofacial growth and development, including genetics, embryology, the normal aging process, and racial and geographic variability of facial form.

FUNDAMENTAL GENETIC CONCEPTS

From the moment of conception, the growth and development of the body is organized by genes. Except for red blood cells, each cell in our body has a nucleus. Within each nucleus are approximately 100,000 genes located on 46 chromosomes. Immediately after conception, these genes begin to determine what types of cells will be formed in our body, where those cells will be located, and what functions they will perform.

Genes are microscopic structures composed of deoxyribonucleic acid (DNA) molecules. Genes, like chromosomes, occur in pairs, and each pair occupies a particular locus, or place, on one of the 23 pairs of chromosomes. Although genes are much too small to be visualized with a light microscope, their molecular structure can be studied using advanced techniques of molecular biology. For detailed descriptions of human genetics and the laboratory methods used to study genes and chromosomes, see Jorde et al. (1995) and Shprintzen (1997).

Malformations

Sometimes errors of genetic structure or function occur. When such mistakes happen, the organism's pre- and postnatal growth and development can be adversely affected. Intrinsic genetic errors produce anomalies, malformations in growth and appearance of body structures. Examples of common malformations include polydactyly (extra fingers or toes), atresia (absence) of the outer ear canal, and syndactyly (fused fingers or toes).

Sequences, Associations, and Syndromes

Sequences result when an individual has a multiple anomaly disorder in which all the anomalies are not related to a single cause (Shprintzen, 1997). Robin sequence is a well known example. In this sequence, it is believed that in-utero deformation of the mandible causes the tongue to remain placed between the developing palatal shelves. The position of the tongue in turn prevents the palatal shelves from assuming a horizontal position and fusing at midline. Failure of fusion results in a large, characteristically U-shaped palatal cleft. Infants born with Robin sequence have a small jaw, cleft palate, and airway obstruction. The infant's tongue, located in a small jaw, cannot maintain a forward position in the airway. The posteriorly positioned tongue falls into the airway and causes airway obstruction while the infant is sleeping.

Associations also produce multiple anomalies in a recurrent pattern. However the etiology or sequential effects which produce associations are currently unknown.

If an individual has multiple anomalies, and all those anomalies have a single cause, then that person is said to have a *syndrome*. If the cause of the syndrome is known, it is classified as a syndrome of *known genesis*; if the cause is unknown, it is called a syndrome of *unknown genesis* (Cohen, 1982). Syndromes of known genesis are further categorized etiologically as chromosomal, genetic, mechanically induced, and teratogenic.

Chromosomal Syndromes

Persons affected by a syndrome often have a characteristic physical appearance, or *phenotype*. Sometimes this phenotype is so distinctive that totally unrelated affected individuals could be mistaken for siblings or genetic relations. Persons with Trisomy 21 (Down's syndrome), for example, can usually be easily identified by their unique facial appearance. In most cases, however, syndromes are diagnosed medically, not visually. Chromosomal syndromes are usually identified by a chromosome analysis, or karyotype.

A *karyotype* is a display of a patient's chromosomes. Chromosomes become visible during the process of cell reproduction. At other times they exist as material called *chromatin* located within a cell's nucleus. As a cell prepares to reproduce itself by dividing, the chromatin in the nucleus becomes organized into 23 pairs of chromosomes. Chromosomes 1 through 22 are known as *autosomes*. Chromosome pair 23 contains the *sex chromosomes*. The X and Y chromosomes are called sex chromosomes because they determine the individual's gender. If the individual is female, she has a pair of X chromosomes. If the individual is male, he has an X and a Y chromosome. Viewed through a light microscope, a pair of chromosomes resembles two V-shaped strings of material (*chromatids*) joined by a central structure, the *centromere* (Figure 2–1). One of the chromatids is usually shorter than the other. In such cases, the shorter chromatid is called the *short*, or p, arm while the longer chromatid is the *long*, or q, arm.

Chromosomes may also be described according to the position of the centromere. Chromosomes with a centrally located centromere are called *metacentric*. If the centromere is near the tip of the p arm, the chromosome is said to be *acrocentric*. In *submetacentric* chromosomes, the centromere is located between the tip of the p arm and the middle of the chromosome.

To prepare a karyotype, living cells are removed from a patient's body and chemically treated to induce cell division. During cell division,

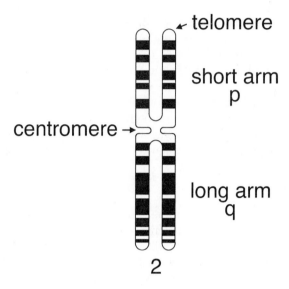

Figure 2–1. Anatomy of a metacentric chromosome. Characteristic banding appears following Giemsa staining.

chromosomes replicate themselves and become visible as aligned pairs. At this point, they are chemically treated again to arrest cell division. The cell nucleus is ruptured, and the chromosome pairs are stained, usually with a chemical called Giemsa. Giemsa staining causes small segments of the chromosomes to appear as light and dark bands (G-bands) on the chromosome's surface. Each chromosome has a characteristic pattern of G-banding. The stained chromosomes are photographed, the photographic image is cut apart, and the photographs of individual chromosomes are numbered and arranged according to length, from longest to shortest, with the sex chromosomes placed in the right-hand corner. The end result of this process is the compilation of a patient's karotype. Although individual genetic anomalies cannot be directly observed from a karyotype, chromosomal errors can be detected by comparing the appearance of the karyotyped chromosomes to normal standards for appearance and G-banding. Table 2–1 summarizes information that can be obtained from a karyotype.

Because chromosomal errors usually involve many individual genes or groups of genes, persons with chromosomal syndromes often have severe multiple anomalies, intellectual and communicative disorders, and craniofacial malformations.

Table 2–1. Information That Can Be Obtained From a Karyotype

Normal male chromosome constitution

Normal female chromosome constitution

Errors of chromosome structure

- Translocations—rearrangement of portions of chromosomes

- Deletions—absence of parts of chromosomes

- Uncommon chromosome aneuploidies: ring chromosomes, dicentric chromosomes, isochromosomes, inversions

Errors of chromosome number

- Monosomy—deletion of an entire chromosome

- Trisomy—presence of an entire extra chromosome

- Polyploidy—presence of one or more complete extra sets of chromosomes

Genetic Syndromes

Changes in sequence of DNA molecules produce genetic variations called mutations. Mutations are responsible for normal genetic variation in traits such as height and eye color, as well as variations that produce single or multiple anomalies. Because of genetic mutation, there can be many possible forms of each of the 100,000 genes. These differing DNA sequences are called *alleles*. A person who has identical alleles on both members of a chromosome pair is said to be *homozygote*. A person with alleles of differing DNA sequence is called *heterozygote*.

Each individual has a specific genetic make up, or *genotype*. Because genes are too small to be visualized, genotypes cannot be visually displayed as chromosomes can. Instead, geneticists study the inheritance patterns of an individual's particular genetic traits to predict the likelihood that these traits will occur in future generations. Figure 2–2 illustrates homozygote and heterozygote configurations and their associated Mendelian inheritance patterns (genetic transmission patterns originally described by Gregor Mendel). After interviewing and observing family members, geneticists often prepare a *pedigree* to illustrate which family members are affected and which are unaffected with a particular genetic disorder.

A pedigree is a kind of family tree that uses symbols to illustrate family relationships, presence of genetic traits, and occurrence of abortions, stillbirths, or twinning. Pedigrees help geneticists determine the type of inheritance pattern for a particular genetic syndrome. Information obtained from a pedigree can also help predict the likelihood of syndrome recurrence in subsequent generations. Figure 2–3 shows the pedigree of a child affected with Waardenburg's syndrome.

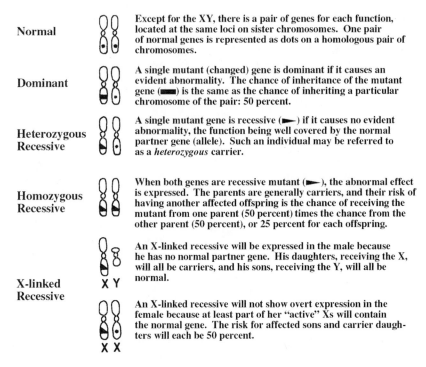

Normal

Except for the XY, there is a pair of genes for each function, located at the same loci on sister chromosomes. One pair of normal genes is represented as dots on a homologous pair of chromosomes.

Dominant

A single mutant (changed) gene is dominant if it causes an evident abnormality. The chance of inheritance of the mutant gene (▬) is the same as the chance of inheriting a particular chromosome of the pair: 50 percent.

Heterozygous Recessive

A single mutant gene is recessive (▶) if it causes no evident abnormality, the function being well covered by the normal partner gene (allele). Such an individual may be referred to as a *heterozygous* carrier.

Homozygous Recessive

When both genes are recessive mutant (▶), the abnormal effect is expressed. The parents are generally carriers, and their risk of having another affected offspring is the chance of receiving the mutant from one parent (50 percent) times the chance from the other parent (50 percent), or 25 percent for each offspring.

X-linked Recessive

An X-linked recessive will be expressed in the male because he has no normal partner gene. His daughters, receiving the X, will all be carriers, and his sons, receiving the Y, will all be normal.

X Y

An X-linked recessive will not show overt expression in the female because at least part of her "active" Xs will contain the normal gene. The risk for affected sons and carrier daughters will each be 50 percent.

X X

Figure 2–2. Homozygous and heterozygous gene pairings and associated inheritance patterns for normal and major mutant genes. (From *Smith's Recognizable Patterns of Human Malformation* [5th ed., p. 716], by K. L. Jones, 1997, Philadelphia: W. B. Saunders Co. Reprinted with permission.)

Because genes continue to control growth and development throughout our lifetime, abnormal genes can have both *long-* and *short-term effects*, as illustrated in the following case study.

Mrs. Jamison was diagnosed with Waardenburg's syndrome (WS) when she was in her late 20s, shortly after her son was born. Her son, Tim, has a profound, congenital, unilateral hearing loss. He also has heterochromia (one blue eye and one brown eye), black hair with a white forelock, and bushy eyebrows extending across his nasal bridge. While discussing Tim's condition with a genetic counselor shortly after Tim's birth, Mrs. Jamison reported that as a child, she had black hair that turned gray when she was 14 years old. Mrs.

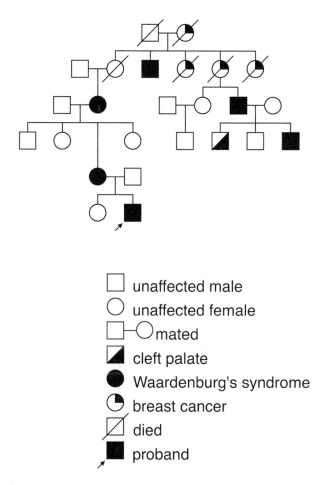

□ unaffected male
○ unaffected female
□─○ mated
◪ cleft palate
● Waardenburg's syndrome
◖ breast cancer
⊘ died
■ proband

Figure 2–3. The proband (person who brought this family under genetic study) in this pedigree is a male child with Waardenburg's syndrome. Note additional family history of breast cancer, unassociated with Waardenburg's syndrome.

Jamison's eyes, which were bright blue in childhood, developed brown patches of color in the irises during adolescence. Mrs. Jamison's hearing was normal until her late 20s, but shortly before Tim's birth, she noticed that understanding conversation in noisy situations was difficult. An audiological evaluation confirmed a mild-to-moderate bilateral sensorineural hearing loss. Since the initial genetic consultation, two of Mrs. Jamison's sisters and three of her maternal uncles have also been diagnosed with WS.

Mrs. Jamison's case illustrates not only the short- and long-term effects of abnormal genes, but the concept of variable genetic expression. A syndrome's phenotypic spectrum includes all possible anomalies that are known to occur in association with that syndrome (in this case, WS). The phenotypic spectrum for WS includes more than 20 anomalies, including broad and high nasal bridge, bushy eyebrows, partial albinism, white forelock, prematurely grey hair, deafness, cleft lip and palate, cardiac anomaly, full lips, and broad mandible. In theory, anyone who has the gene for WS could experience the entire phenotypic spectrum; in reality this seldom occurs. Mrs. Jamison's phenotype included only problems of eye and hair pigmentation early in life, followed by hearing loss in adulthood. Her son's phenotype included pigmentation problems, unusual facial features, and a serious congenital hearing loss. Variable genetic expression can delay syndrome diagnosis, as it did in Mrs. Jamison's family, and affect long-term treatment options.

As clinicians, we can observe the effects of abnormal genes as expressed in a patient's physical appearance and behavioral characteristics (phenotype). Phenotypes are diagnostically useful because in many cases they are so distinct as to make the presence of a particular syndrome immediately recognizable. Once a syndrome has been diagnosed, the phenotypic spectrum suggests a plan for diagnostic testing, treatment, and patient counseling.

Chromosomal and genetic syndromes produce anomalies because they alter an individual's normal genetic makeup, sometimes from the moment of conception. Because chromosomal and genetic syndromes can be inherited, they have the potential to affect not only the persons born with the syndrome, but future generations of individuals born to affected persons.

Craniofacial anomalies can occur even if an individual's genetic makeup is normal. To understand how mechanical forces and teratogens affect developing individuals, we must first understand some basic principles of embryology.

UNDERSTANDING EMBRYOLOGY

Most people enjoy looking at photographs of babies and children and observing the physical changes that occur during childhood. When we observe a photograph of a newborn baby, we are actually seeing a photograph of a nine-month-old baby, assuming the child was the product of a normal, nine-month pregnancy. We seldom consider what that baby looked like during its nine months in utero; even less often do we see in-

utero photographs. To visualize how an individual looks from conception to birth, we must rely on information gained from embryological
studies. Although embryology technically means the study of embryos,
the term is used in a more general sense to describe the study of
embryos, fetuses, and prenatal development. It is beyond the scope of
this text to review all aspects of embryology and prenatal development.
Only basic definitions and concepts critical to the understanding of
craniofacial anomalies will be mentioned here. For in-depth descriptions
of embryological development, consult Moore and Persaud (1998) and
Sperber (1998).

Embryological Development

Embryological development extends from conception to the eighth
week in utero. During this time, growth takes place rapidly and is
described in stages, beginning with stage 1 at fertilization and ending at
stage 23 on day 56. At the end of eight weeks, the beginnings of all major
structures are present, although only the heart and circulatory system
are functioning.

After the embryonic period ends, the fetal period begins, and the
developing individual is called a *fetus*. The fetal period extends from the
ninth week of life until birth. During this time, previously formed structures differentiate, grow, and begin to function. Body growth and weight
gain also occur throughout this period.

Development of the Head and Neck

By the fourth week in utero, the human embryo resembles a curved
structure (Figure 2–4) that measures about 4 mm from crown to rump
(about the size of half a watermelon seed). The major structures visible
at this time include placodes, somites, and the pharyngeal apparatus.

Placodes

Placodes are thickened areas of embryonic ectoderm from which senso-
ry organs will arise. Nasal, otic, and optic placodes will eventually contribute to the development of the nose, ears, and eyes respectively.

Somites

Somites are paired masses of cells that begin to develop in the embryonic paraxial mesoderm about day 20. They first appear in what will
become the occipital region of the head and continue to develop cau-

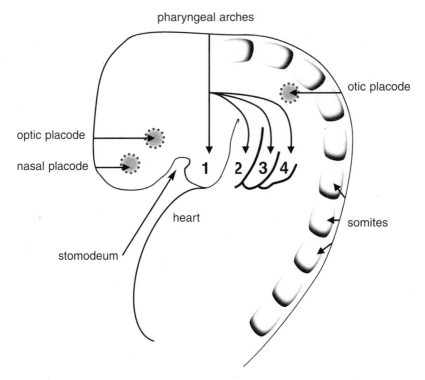

Figure 2–4. Left lateral view of a 28-day-old human embryo showing initial development of placodes, somites, and pharyngeal arches.

dally until 42 to 44 pairs ultimately appear on either side of the neural tube. The appearance of somites is so distinct during the fourth and fifth week of life that the number of somites can be used to calculate the embryo's age. Somites eventually become the structures of the axial skeleton, the associated musculature, and the dermis of the skin.

Pharyngeal Apparatus

The pharyngeal apparatus consists of pharyngeal arches, pharyngeal pouches, pharyngeal grooves, and pharyngeal membranes (Moore & Persaud, 1998). Structures of the head and neck arise from this apparatus.

Pharyngeal arches. Pharyngeal arches are visible as a series of bilateral swellings on the lateral surfaces of the embryo. They are numbered craniocaudally from one to six. Pharyngeal arch five is sometimes absent; in any case, arches four and six eventually merge to collectively form what will become laryngeal structures.

Each pharyngeal arch contains an artery, a bar of cartilage, a cranial nerve, and a muscular component. Table 2–2 shows the derivatives of structures of the pharyngeal apparatus. Notice particularly that the first pharyngeal arch, also called the mandibular arch, has two enlarged areas: the maxillary prominence, or the process that will eventually become the maxilla, zygomatic bone, and squamous part of the temporal bone; and the mandibular prominence that will form the mandible. The first arch is extremely important to head, neck, and middle-ear development.

Table 2–2. Derivatives and Innervation of Pharyngeal Arches

Pharyngeal Arch	Cranial Nerve	Muscles	Skeletal Structures
Mandibular I	Trigeminal V Mandibular division	• Muscles of mastication (temporalis, masseter, medial and lateral pterygoids) • Mylohyoid • Anterior belly of digastric • Tensor veli palatini • Temporalis muscle	• Malleus, incus, portion of mandible • Anterior ligament of malleus • Sphenomandibular ligament
Hyoid 2	Facial VII	• Muscles of facial expression (buccinator, frontalis auricularis, platysma, orbicularis oris, and oculi) • Posterior belly of digastric • Stylohyoid • Stapedius	• Stapes • Styloid process • Lesser horn and upper portion of body of hyoid bone
3	Glossopharyngeal IX	Stylopharyngeus	• Greater horn and lower portion of body of hyoid bone
4, 5, 6	Vagus X Superior laryngeal branch to 4th arch Recurrent laryngeal	Cricothyroid • Levator palatini • Pharyngeal constrictors • Intrinsic muscles of larynx (thyroarytenoids, lateral cricoarytenoids, posterior cricoarytenoids, interarytenoids)	• Laryngeal cartilages (thyroid, cricoid, arytenoid)

Pharyngeal pouches, grooves, and membranes. Pharyngeal arches are separated from one another on the embryo's external surface by pharyngeal grooves and internally by pharyngeal pouches. These deep fissures are also numbered craniocaudally. Pouches and grooves are spaces, not solid structures, that contribute to development of cavities and spaces such as the ear canal, middle-ear cavity, and tonsilar crypts. Table 2–3 shows derivatives of pharyngeal pouches, grooves, and membranes.

Pharyngeal membranes are solid structures that form where epithelial cells of pouches and grooves adjoin one another. The first pharyngeal membrane is the only membrane that survives to become a structure in the adult human. This membrane forms the tympanic membrane that separates the outer from the middle ear.

Facial Development

Facial development occurs between the fourth and eighth week of life. In the fourth week, structures that will become the face begin to become organized around a central opening, the *stomodeum*. The development of

Table 2–3. Derivatives of Pharyngeal Pouches, Grooves, and Membranes

Embryonic Structure	Adult Structure
First pharyngeal pouch	Tympanic cavity Mastoidantrium Auditory tube Eustachian tube
Second pharyngeal pouch	Tonsilar fossa Surface epithelium and lining of tonsillar crypts
Third pharyngeal pouch	Inferior parathyroid gland Thymus
Fourth pharyngeal pouch	Superior parathyroid gland
Pharyngeal grooves	
First pharyngeal groove Remaining grooves are obliterated as the neck develops	External auditory meatus
Pharyngeal membrane	
First pharyngeal membrane	Tympanic membrane

embryological structures, including facial structures, is easier to learn if we remember that the human body is organized bilaterally. Most major external features (eyes, ears, limbs, digits) and many internal features (kidneys, lungs, bones of axial skeleton, cranial and spinal nerves, hemispheres of the cerebral and cerebellar cortex) occur in pairs. In most of us, these paired structures are approximately the same size and shape. This identical bilateral appearance is called *bilateral symmetry* and is an important component of what constitutes "normal" craniofacial appearance. Bilateral symmetry also makes understanding embryological development easier, particularly when considering the formation of the human face.

The Facial Primordia

If we look at the "face" of a 4-week-old embryo (Figure 2–5), we will see five enlarged areas of tissue surrounding the stomodeum. The stomodeum opens into an area that will eventually be the oral cavity. The five surrounding tissue areas begin to form when neural crest cells migrate to the stomodeal area from the neural folds early in the fourth week of life. Neural crest cells are the original source for many of the ligaments, connective tissues, cartilages, and bones of the face and oral cavity.

Imagine that the stomodeal opening is a clock face. The area that occupies the space above and around the area from approximately 10:00 to 2:00 is called the *frontonasal prominence*. The embryo's forebrain is developing behind this centrally located prominence, and nasal placodes are forming bilaterally on its external surface.

The areas of tissue located at 9:00 to 10:00 and 2:00 to 3:00 are called *maxillary prominences*. These are the parts of the first pharyngeal arches

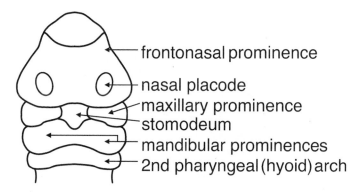

Figure 2–5. Facial primordia of a human embryo at 4 weeks.

that will become three major bones of the midface: the maxilla, the zygomatic bone, and the squamous portion of the temporal bone.

The *mandibular prominences* occupy the remaining area of the clock, from 3:00 to 9:00. These paired prominences are also part of the first pharyngeal arch and will eventually form such structures as the mandible and ossicular chain. Collectively, then, the *facial primordia* consists of a frontonasal prominence, a pair of maxillary prominences, and a pair of mandibular prominences.

Nasal Development

By the end of the fourth week, nasal placodes have become organized bilaterally on the frontonasal process. The edges of the placodes develop elevated areas of tissue: the *medial* and *lateral nasal prominences* (Figure 2–6). The placodes themselves have formed depressions (nasal pits) that eventually become the nostrils (nares) and nasal cavities of the nose. A groove (nasolacrimal groove) separates the lateral nasal prominences from the maxillary prominences.

External Ears

During the fifth week, the external ears begin to develop in what is initially the region of the neck (Figure 2–7). Six small areas of mesenchymal

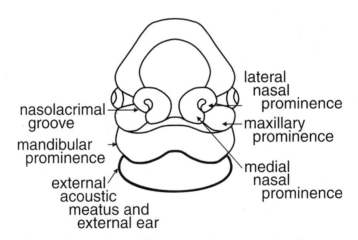

Figure 2–6. ''Face'' of a human embryo at approximately five and one-half weeks. Note that maxilla, mandible, nares, and external ear are developing rapidly.

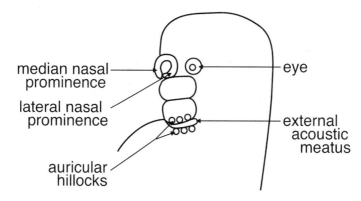

Figure 2–7. Left lateral view of a human embryo showing ear development at approximately 5 weeks.

tissue form around the first pharyngeal groove. As the mandible develops, these six *auricular hillocks* are elevated up the side of the head to the level of the eyes. The auricular hillocks will eventually become the auricles of the outer ear.

The Intermaxillary Segment and Primary Palate

By the end of the sixth week, the maxillary prominences begin to merge with the lateral nasal prominences along the nasolacrimal groove. The medial nasal prominences merge with one another and with the maxillary and lateral nasal prominences from the seventh through the tenth weeks. As a result of the merging of the medial nasal and maxillary prominences, the *intermaxillary segment* is formed (Figure 2–8). The intermaxillary segment is an important area of tissue that will eventually produce the *philtrum* of the upper lip, the *premaxilla* of the maxilla, and the *alveolar ridge*. Collectively the upper lip, premaxilla, and alveolar ridge are called the *primary palate*.

The Secondary Palate

The secondary palate consists of the hard and soft palates from the posterior border of the premaxilla to the end of the uvula. The secondary palate begins to develop early in the sixth week from two internal maxillary structures called lateral palatine processes (palatal shelves). Figure 2–9 shows the relationship of the palatal shelves to the tongue, the nasal septum and the mandibular prominences during the sixth to twelfth

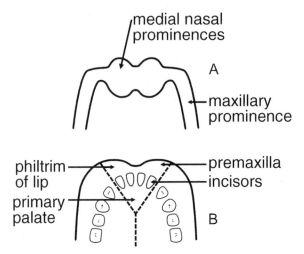

Figure 2–8. Horizontal section of maxillary process at approximately 5 weeks (**A**). Darkened central area represents fused medial nasal prominences. (**B**) shows location of primary palate, including philtrum of lip and premaxilla, and future location of teeth. Dotted lines indicate points of fusion between primary and secondary palates: Note that tooth development and location may be affected if primary and secondary palates fail to fuse properly.

weeks. The mandible opens as it develops and creates space in the oral cavity (Figure 2–9A). This space allows the tongue to become relocated from the nasal to the oral cavity (Figure 2–9B). As the tongue descends, the palatal shelves assume a horizontal position and fuse from front to back along the midline during the eighth to tenth week of development (Figure 2–9C). The palatal shelves also fuse with the posterior borders of the primary palate and between the ninth and twelfth week with the nasal septum while the maxillary prominences produce the lateral parts of the upper lip and most of the maxilla. We can best appreciate the contribution of the pharyngeal apparatus to facial development if we compare the embryonic face (see Figure 2–6) to the fully developed face of an adult (Figure 2–10).

Environmental Factors

Although genetic and chromosomal malformations can be manifested during the embryonic and fetal periods, genetically normal individuals can also experience problems during prenatal development. Environ-

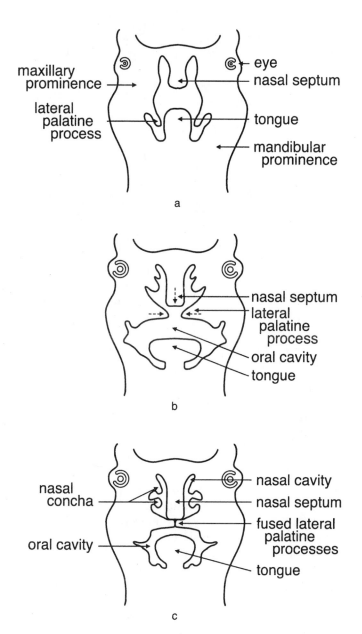

Figure 2–9. Coronal view of development of the secondary palate. Note that tongue initially occupies the space between developing palatal shelves (**A**). Tongue descends as mandible develops (**B**), and palatal shelves fuse with one another and with nasal septum (**C**).

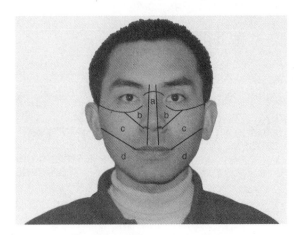

Figure 2–10. Location of former embryonic structures in a fully developed adult face: **A.** Medial nasal prominence. **B.** Lateral nasal prominence. **C.** Maxillary prominence. **D.** Mandibular prominence.

mental factors can interfere with normal prenatal growth to produce two types of syndromes: mechanically induced and teratogenically induced.

Mechanically Induced Syndromes

When outside forces change the process of growth and development, either pre- or postnatally, the resulting anomalies are called *deformations*. Deformations may occur when two or more fetuses share a confined space in utero, for example. Other times, the mother's uterus is malformed, and the cranium, limbs, or facial features of her developing baby may be compressed into an abnormal shape. Deformations can also occur after birth if the child's movement or body position is restricted for long periods of time. Physicians often recommend that babies be left in a supine sleeping position to avoid sudden infant death syndrome. It is increasingly common to see infants who have acquired a flattened occipital skull shape after being restricted to sleeping in this recommended position for several months. Because deformations do not involve changes to genes or chromosomes, they are not transmissible to future generations. Deformations can often be successfully corrected or modified postnatally through surgical or orthopedic management. For a detailed explanation of deformation patterns and an overview of the mechanics of growth and development consult the works of Smith (1981) and Enlow and Hans (1996).

Teratogenic Syndromes

Sometimes the process of growth and development is altered by the effects of environmental agents called teratogens. Although teratogens are traditionally defined as agents that can produce a congenital anomaly (Persaud, 1990), we must remember that our bodies continue to grow postnatally. Although some periods of development are more vulnerable to the effects of teratogens than others, our bodies remain at risk to the effects of teratogens throughout our lifetimes. The effect of tetracycline on tooth development is a good example of how teratogens can affect both pre- and postnatal growth. Teeth continue developing from 18 weeks prenatally to 16 years postnatally. This means that maternal ingestion of tetracycline by a pregnant woman may cause her child's teeth to be discolored or to have dysplastic tooth enamel. On the other hand, a child who ingests tetracycline postnatally may also develop discolored enamel of the permanent dentition because tooth development continues into adolescence.

Environmental factors (teratogens) account for 7 to 10% of congenital anomalies (Moore & Persaud, 1998). Known teratogens include chemicals, drugs, infections, and high levels of radiation. The potential effect of a teratogen depends on timing, dosage, and genotype of the embryo (Moore & Persaud, 1998). Timing is particularly important. A *critical period* is that time during which a developing tissue or organ is most vulnerable to the effects of a particular teratogen. Figure 2–11 illustrates critical periods of human development with respect to teratogenic effects. Notice that specific sites such as eyes, heart, limbs, and brain are especially vulnerable to teratogenic effects. Systems or body parts that develop simultaneously may be simultaneously affected by teratogens. During the 1950s, for example, an outbreak of rubella in the United States caused many children to be born deaf, blind, and mentally retarded. The rubella virus is a teratogen that can cause serious malformations or death if contracted by a developing embryo. The eyes, ears, and brain develop simultaneously and are particularly vulnerable to teratogenic effects. Those children who were exposed to the rubella virus in utero during a critical time of development for the eyes, ears, and central nervous system were therefore born with multiple congenital malformations.

Children exposed to rubella or other teratogens during the first two weeks in utero, on the other hand, are likely to have an "all or nothing" response. During this time, the embryo is either able to overcome the effects of exposure to a teratogen, or the embryo is so severely affected by the teratogen that it cannot survive.

By learning the principles of embryological organization and growth, clinicians can more easily visualize developmental relationships between seemingly unrelated body parts. Understanding relationships of *timing, origin,* and *proximity* helps us to ask appropriate diagnostic questions and to draw accurate diagnostic conclusions based on observations of a patient's physical appearance.

As illustrated in Figure 2–11, several major organ systems have simultaneous critical development periods, times during which they are particularly vulnerable to teratogenic effects. Knowing when these critical developmental periods occur assists physicians in diagnosing the etiology of a problem, or conversely, to pinpoint the time of teratogenic insult when the etiology is already known.

Many embryological structures *originate* from a common source. Knowing the embryological relationship between structures of a common origin enables us to understand relationships between externally visible anatomical structures and associated structures that are not readily observable. We know, for example, that the mandible and the middle ear originate from the same location (the first pharyngeal arch). This allows us to make diagnostic assumptions about the development, structure, and function of the middle ear based on the external appearance of the mandible.

The growth and development of some embryological structures depends on shared *proximity* during development. Structures that are located near one another may affect one another's growth and development, even if both structures have different embryological origins. Understanding proximity of embryological structures allows us to recognize diagnostic relationships between seemingly unrelated areas of the human body. The heart and the vocal folds, for example, are two structures with unrelated origins. Normal vocal fold function postnatally depends in part on the structure of the heart, because of an embryological relationship that begins during the simultaneous development of cranial nerve X and the heart. Knowing this early relationship helps us understand why children with congenital heart problems often have left vocal fold paralysis and an accompanying voice disorder.

UNDERSTANDING POSTNATAL GROWTH AND AGING

When we observe a patient's craniofacial appearance, we basically want to know if that appearance is normal or atypical. Most of us have used commercially marketed or in-house oral-facial screening examinations to help make such determinations. Although oral-facial screening protocols provide an ideal beginning for the process of craniofacial observation, they have limitations. Generic screening protocols provide

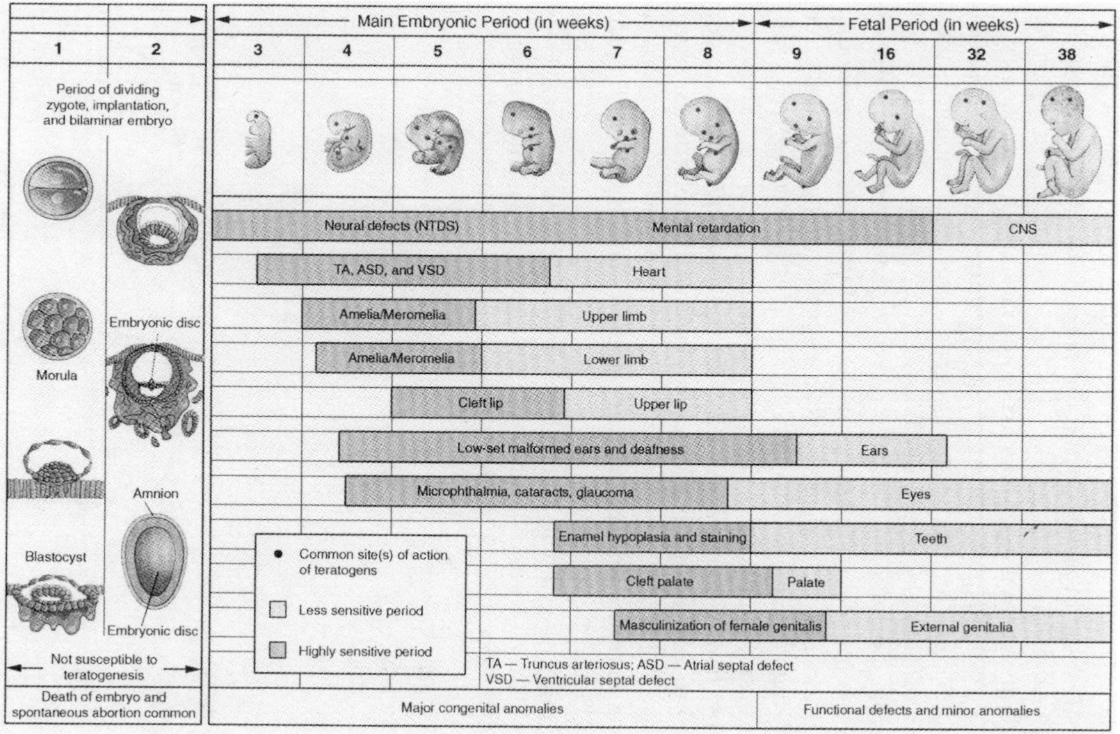

Figure 2–11. Effects of teratogens during critical periods of human prenatal development (*From The Developing Human* [6th ed.] by K.L Moore and T.V.N. Persaud, 1998, p. 182. Philadelphia: W. B. Saunders Co. Reprinted with permission.)

guidelines for observing basic craniofacial appearance but most do not include guidelines for observing normal age, gender, and racially related differences, although these differences are sometimes substantial.

When using such protocols, we must adjust our observational expectations to our patient's age, gender, and racial background. We will begin by considering what constitutes "normal" facial features for children and for adults.

As humans, the shape of our skulls and faces are determined in part by the shape and growth pattern of our developing brains. Enlow (1990), describes three basic skull shapes common to human beings: *dolichocephalic*, *brachycephalic*, and *mesocephalic* (Figure 2–12). Dolichocephalic and brachycephalic shapes represent extremes in skull appearance, while mesocephalic lies somewhere between the two. Although normal variations in brain and skull shape have no effect on intellectual capacity, they do have substantial effect on midface development, profile appearance, and molar relationships.

Individuals with a brachycephalic head shape have a round, wide brain; a prognathic profile; and an Angle Class III molar relationship. Persons with a dolichocephalic head shape, on the other hand, usually have long, narrow brains; retrognathic profiles; and Angle Class II molar relationships (Enlow, 1990).

As in the developing embryo, craniofacial appearance changes as an individual grows and develops. With the exception of embryological changes, the craniofacial changes that occur in childhood are the most dramatic.

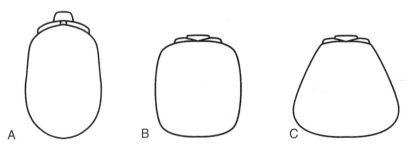

Figure 2–12. Normal human skull shapes. **A.** Dolichocephalic, a form common in Caucasian and African individuals. **B.** Brachycephalic, frequently noted in Oriental persons and some female Caucasian individuals. **C.** Mesocephalic, a shape that can occur in any race.

Age Related Changes in Craniofacial Appearance

Prepubertal Child

Newborn infants of all races usually begin life with a brachycephalic skull shape that becomes substantially modified as the child matures. A review of some basic principles of age-related growth changes explains why this is so.

Although a newborn baby has a fully formed body, he or she continues to grow and change in appearance throughout life. Such growth is influenced by a number of interrelated factors, including genetic inheritance, nutritional intake, development of the airway, and the interaction between growth patterns of individual anatomical structures. Growth of craniofacial structures occurs in spurts rather than as a slow, steady process. The brain, teeth, facial muscles, and sinuses grow at different rates and develop at different times during childhood. Their growth (or lack of growth) significantly impacts the development of surrounding structures.

When we observe a typical baby's appearance, we notice that the child has a large head with large eyes that are positioned prominently in a small face. The proportions of the baby's face are initially dictated by rapid brain growth. The baby's face appears small in part because the brain is large relative to the face beneath it and because the baby's mandible is small. To some extent, mandibular growth depends on the eruption of primary and secondary dentition, neither of which has occurred in the infant. The child's eyes, on the other hand, develop simultaneously with the nervous system and are almost as large in the infant's face as they will be when the infant becomes an adult.

Table 2–4 summarizes the normal facial appearance of a prepubertal child. Guidelines for prepubertal facial appearance are essentially identical for boys and girls but differ slightly according to racial background, as we will see.

Essentially, a young child's face has a proportionately large cranium with a convex forehead, chubby cheeks, a small mouth, and a small chin. The nose is usually short and appears concave in profile. The nasal bridge is low and broad. Because the nasal bridge is almost as large as it will be in adulthood, the child's eyes appear wide set and larger than they actually are. In many children, especially Asian and African children, the low nasal bridge allows the overlying skin to drape in folds across the inner corners of the eye (*epicanthal folds*). Epicanthal folds remain a normal facial feature for Asian adults because low nasal bridges are a normal facial feature for adult Asians. Although Asian persons retain epicanthal folds throughout life, most Caucasians and persons of African descent lose this feature after the airway and the nasal bridge develop completely.

Table 2–4. Normal Facial Appearance of Prepubertal Child of Either Gender

Head

- Shape is brachycephalic: wide, vertically short, rounded
- Lower two-thirds of face appears relatively flat; cheekbones are prominent, and cheeks may be chubby
- All six fontaneles are completely closed by 18 months
- Forehead profile appears noticeably convex and upright
- Head appears to sit directly on shoulders of very young child
- Prepubertal child appears to have slender neck beneath large head

Mandible

- Infant chin appears very small
- Infant mandible appears short and pointed
- Primary and secondary dentition not apparent in infant
- Mandible grows larger as dentition develops

Eyes

- Appear blue in newborn regardless of race or gender
- Appear wide set because of low nasal bridge
- Appear large and bulging in contrast to small midface and lower face
- Epicanthal folds may be present as normal feature in young child regardless of race or gender

Nose

- Infant nose appears short, round, "snubbed"
- Infant nose has concave, low, broad nasal bridge
- Infant nares can be seen in a face-on view

Mouth

- Infant mouth appears small in proportion to rest of face

Ears

- Infant ears appear low set compared to placement of adult ears

---

Newborns and infants appear to have almost no neck. The baby's neck develops as the child begins to walk upright and as the child's airway changes position from the horizontal configuration of the newborn to the vertical airway of the older child. We can appreciate the still relatively horizontal location of laryngeal structures in very young children by observing the epiglottis that is often visible in the oral cavity, just posterior to the back of the tongue.

In addition to airway development, other major craniofacial changes occurring during childhood include closure of fontanels, eruption of primary and permanent dentition, enlargement of the facial sinuses, growth of the mandible, enlargement of the midface bones, and development of the chin.

Puberty to Young Adulthood

Puberty marks the time when gender related changes in facial structure appear. These changes are most noticeable in males, particularly in the nasal region. On the whole, males have a larger overall body size than females, including larger lungs and bigger muscles. Larger bodies require larger airways to conduct an adequate supply of oxygen to body tissues. They need larger noses to supply air to larger airways. This is one reason why males generally have larger, more prominent noses than females have. Adult males often have a dolichocephalic head shape, one with a long nose, protrusive features, and an angular appearance. Adult females, on the other hand, are likely to retain the brachycephalic head shape of infancy with its wide, flat face and small nose.

Normal facial features of male and female adults are summarized in Table 2–5. Remember that these features are *guidelines* of normal appearance, based on the craniofacial structure of large populations of people. A female who has a large, protrusive nose, dolichocephalic head shape, protruding brow ridges, and a large mouth may look masculine, but her facial appearance is still considered normal. Likewise, a male with small nose, flat face, small brows, and brachycephalic head shape may appear to have feminine facial features. The appearance of masculine facial features in a woman or feminine facial features in a man in the absence of other abnormality should be considered normal variability in facial appearance, rather than an indication of a syndrome or craniofacial malformation.

By age 18 for both genders, the mandible has completely developed, and the majority of permanent dentition has erupted. Although the majority of craniofacial development has taken place by early adulthood, the face continues to change throughout life as a result of normal aging. Age-related change in facial appearance is an important topic, but one that is too extensive to be addressed here. Remember, however, that the craniofacial complex continues to change throughout a lifetime and that you may be called upon to distinguish between normal age-related changes and craniofacial anomalies in older patients.

Table 2–5. Normal Facial Appearance of Male and Female Adults

Female Face

- Head shape often brachycephalic, but may be dolichocephalic or a combination of brachycephalic and dolichocephalic
- Forehead profile appears bulbous and upright
- Supraorbital ridges are less prominent than in male face
- Cheekbones appear more visible because of upright forehead
- Face looks flatter, wider, more delicate than male face

Male Face

- Head shape likely to be dolichocephalic, but may be brachycephalic, or a combination of brachycephalic and dolichocephalic
- Forehead profile is sloping
- Supraorbital ridges are very prominent
- Eyes appear deep set because of protrusive supraorbital ridges
- Face looks deep, with coarser features than female face

Female Nose

- Appears smaller, thinner, less prominent than male nose
- Appears less protrusive than male nose
- Entire nose appears straight to concave in profile
- Tip of nose appears rounded in profile with upward tilt
- Nares may be visible in face-on view

Male Nose

- Appears large, prominent, and protrusive
- Looks longer and wider than female nose
- Tip of nose may be pointed with flaring nostrils
- Appears straight to convex in profile

Racial Background and Craniofacial Appearance

Health care professionals are often placed in the position of providing service to patients whose racial background differs from their own. After a lifetime of observing people of our own ethnic background, most of us have become familiar with what is acceptable "normal" appearance in people "like us." For several generations, standards for normal growth and development in the United States have been standards based on studies of Caucasians. This situation has occurred in part because Caucasians were the most readily available population to study and in part because anatomical studies of specific racial populations were considered discriminatory. Comparative research on racial differences (if any) in craniofacial appearance is needed if we are to provide accurate health care to diverse populations. If significant differences exist, we need to know what they are and what their implications for patient treatment might be. In the meantime, we must try to distinguish between normal and abnormal craniofacial appearance no matter what the race of the person we are observing.

Table 2–6 summarizes the variability of facial appearance among racial groups. Notice that many of the features that contribute to unique racial appearance are internal. In such cases, we are likely to observe the *results* of racial differences, rather than the differences themselves. The significantly broader mandibular ramus of adult persons of African descent is such an example. Without observing cephalometric photographs of a given individual, we are not likely to know the dimensions of the mandibular ramus or of any other facial bone. By observing a patient's occlusal relationship, however, a highly skilled observer can visually recognize the results of the presence of a broad mandibular ramus: labially tipped maxillary incisors with resulting bimaxillary protrusion (Enlow, 1990).

Remember that despite a given individual's head shape, much intraracial variability in facial appearance exists. Figure 2–13 illustrates facial variability in four individuals of Asian background. In reality, there is also considerable interracial blending among ethnic groups. Therefore, use guidelines for normal racial appearance *as* guidelines, general trends that are diagnostically useful when viewed in the perspective of a patient's overall facial appearance.

Geographic Origin and Craniofacial Appearance

Geographic origin of an ethnic group also affects facial appearance, particularly in the areas of skin and eye pigmentation and nasal configuration. People whose ancestors originated from cold climates often have light colored hair, pale skin, blue or light colored eyes, and long, thin noses. Melanin, the pigment that darkens in response to sunlight, protects our bodies from sun-induced damage. People living in cold climates receive less intense exposure to sunlight and so do not need extensive pigmentation for protection. They *do* need a way to warm cold air before it reaches the surface of the lungs. Long thin noses have large internal surfaces with an abundant blood supply for warming and humidifying cold, dry air.

Table 2–6. Racial Differences in Facial Appearance of Adults

Caucasian (sometimes called white) Appearance

- Head shape of male is usually dolichocephalic. Head shape of female is usually brachycephalic, but either gender may have brachycephalic, dolichocephalic or some shape in between
- Brain volume same as Asian or African, but shape is usually narrow
- Upper face is protrusive and lower face more retrusive than other groups
- Retrognathic profile common
- Mandibular ramus may be broad, but not as broad as African
- Cheekbones may appear less prominent because of upper face and midface protrusion
- Class II malocclusion is frequent

Asian (sometimes called Oriental) Appearance

- Head shape often brachycephalic because brain is round and horizontally short
- In profile, forehead appears bulbous and upright
- Eyebrow ridges are less protrusive than other groups
- Frontal sinus is small
- Nasal bridge is low
- Epicanthal folds are present
- Profile often appears orthognathic
- Cheekbones prominent in contrast to less protrusive upper face and midface
- Eyes appear wide set because nasal bridge is low
- Class III malocclusion and prognathic mandible may be present

African (sometimes called Black or Negroid) Appearance

- Head shape likely to be dolichocephalic
- Nasomaxillary complex may be vertically long
- Upper part of face less protrusive than Caucasian
- Forehead more upright and bulbous than Caucasian
- Nasal bridge lower than Caucasian; nose flatter, wider, less protrusive
- Cheekbones appear prominent
- Mandibular ramus significantly broader than Caucasian
- Class II malocclusion may be present

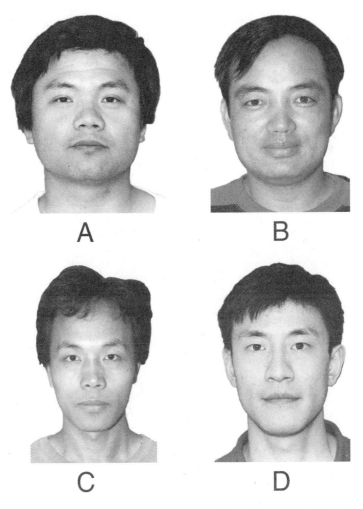

Figure 2–13. Normal facial variability among four Chinese males. Person A has brachycephalic skull shape typical of many Asians. Individual B has a somewhat mesocephalic appearance, while persons C and D exhibit a more dolichocephalic appearance. All subjects have epicanthal folds and broad nasal bridges, although not to an equal degree.

By contrast, people living in hot, humid climates need the extensive sun protection provided by increased melanin. This results in darker hair, skin, and eye color. People whose ancestors originated in such climates typically have broad, flat noses because there is no need for modifying temperature or humidity of air entering the lungs in such environments. The geographic origin of a particular ethnic group, then, may be one reason for variability in nasal size and shape between ethnic groups (Carey & Steegmann, 1981).

Postnatal growth of the human face is an enormously complex topic that cannot be discussed in depth in this text. For a thorough explanation of pre- and postnatal craniofacial growth processes, see Enlow and Hans (1996). For a collection of anthropomorphic measures of normal anatomical growth, consult Kent and Vorperian (1995).

SUMMARY

During a diagnostic session, we have the opportunity to observe results of the interaction of genetic, embryological, and environmental influences on a given individual's craniofacial development. As our knowledge of these subjects increases, we can become more skilled observers. Skilled observers are persons who have learned how to recognize the effects of genetic, embryological, and environmental influences, and how to make differential diagnoses accordingly. This chapter has provided a general overview of the genetic, embryological, racial and age-related changes that influence craniofacial development. We now need to learn how to observe, what to observe, how to extract diagnostic information from our observations, and how to proceed with diagnostic recommendations.

REFERENCES

Carey, J. W., & Steegmann, A. T. (1981). Human nasal protrusion, latitude and climate. *American Journal of Physiological Anthropology, 56,* 313–319.

Cohen, M. M., Jr. (1982). *The child with multiple birth defects.* New York: Raven Press.

Enlow, D. H. (1990). *Facial growth.* Philadelphia: W. B. Saunders Co.

Enlow, D. H., & Hans, M. G. (1996). *Essentials of facial growth.* Philadelphia: W. B. Saunders Co.

Jorde, L. B., Carey, J. C., & White, R. L. (1995). *Medical genetics.* St. Louis, MO: Mosby.

Kent, R. D., & Vorperian, H. K. (1995). *Development of the craniofacial-oral-laryngeal anatomy: A review.* San Diego, CA: Singular Publishing Group, Inc.

Moore, K. L., & Persaud, T. V. N. (1998). *The developing human* (6th ed.). Philadelphia: W. B. Saunders Co.

Persaud, T. V. N. (1990). *Environmental causes of human birth defects.* Springfield, MO: Charles C. Thomas.

Shprintzen, R. J. (1997). *Genetics, syndromes, and communication disorders.* San Diego, CA: Singular Publishing Group.

Smith, D. W. (1981). *Recognizable patterns of human deformation.* Philadelphia: W. B. Saunders Co.

Sperber, D. H. (1998). *Craniofacial embryology.* Woburn, MA: Butterworth-Heinemann.

CHAPTER 3

LEARNING TO OBSERVE: COLLECTING INFORMATION

Students often believe that diagnosis is the first step in the rehabilitation process. Although accurate diagnosis is essential to accurate treatment, it is really the *second* step; rehabilitation begins when someone recognizes that a problem exists.

Although the complete diagnostic process has several components (patient interviews, appropriate specific testing, consultation with colleagues, recommendations, referrals, and family counseling), this chapter will address the aspects of clinical observation. To do that, we need to understand what clinical observation is.

In some diagnostic settings, hastily performed, cursory intraoral examinations are routine practice and constitute what many professionals regard as the "clinical observation" part of diagnosis. Although intraoral exams are important and should remain part of the diagnostic process, the art of clinical observation is far more complex. Clinical observation is a systematic way of observing the whole patient, a method of collecting, analyzing, and interpreting visual, tactile, and auditory observations. This chapter presents guidelines for collecting visual information using clinical observation techniques. These techniques can be used as initial steps preceding diagnostic referral, or *in addition* to the routine intraoral examination component of a formal diagnostic session.

WHAT CAN I LEARN FROM VISUAL OBSERVATIONS?

As a trained observer, you can use information obtained from visual observations to:

- identify normal patients
- assess a patient's state of health
- identify patients at risk for genetic problems
- compile a patient's phenotype
- reassess a patient's appearance following surgical or orthodontic treatment
- prepare a long-term treatment plan
- collect research data

Let's examine some of these benefits more closely.

Recognizing "Normal"

Systematic observation of the patient as a whole, and of the patient's craniofacial complex in particular, allows clinicians to compare a patient to normative standards appropriate to that person's age, gender, and racial background when such standards exist.

When no generally accepted standards are available, as is the case for some ethnic groups and for biracial individuals, we must rely on information from specific research studies or on generally accepted ideas of what constitutes "normal." Unfortunately, widely accepted standards may be diagnostically misleading, at least during a cursory observation. A recent study comparing normal black African newborns to black African newborns with Down's syndrome (DS) emphasizes the way in which lack of specific ethnic normative data and failure to observe the entire child may be affecting early detection of Down's syndrome (DS) in black children in East Africa. In seeking to determine why there is an apparent low prevalence of DS in black African children, Christianson, Kromberg, and Viljoen (1995) compared craniofacial features of 40 black neonates with DS to 50 black neonates without DS. Results were then compared to previous studies of Caucasian newborns with and without DS. The authors discovered that craniofacial features of the black African newborns with DS were very similar in appearance to those of normal black African newborns. Craniofacial features of newborn DS Caucasians, however, differed markedly from their normal counterparts. Flat facial profiles and epicanthal folds are common diagnostic indications of DS in both black and Caucasian neonates. The authors suggest that when such features are present in Caucasian infants, they are often considered "different" enough to alert medical professionals to the possibility of a genetic problem. In black infants, however, epicanthal folds, low nasal bridge, and flat facial profile occur so often that they constitute "normal" appearance and generally excite little concern among medical personnel. Therefore, craniofacial anomalies that cause diagnostic concern in Caucasian infants may go unnoticed in black infants because these features approximate what is considered "normal" craniofacial appearance for black children. This study emphasizes the continued need for careful visual observation of the entire patient, as well as a need for specific age-, gender-, and race-appropriate normative standards.

Most of the observational techniques we will learn are informal guidelines for "normal," rather than absolute measures. Absolute measures do exist, however, for specific features in specific populations, and there may be times when we wish to use them.

In cases where informal visual assessment is not sufficient (collecting data for research studies, for example) it may be necessary to measure the patient's craniofacial structures to confirm that visual observations are accurate. Ear size, head circumference, and eye placement are particularly difficult to visually access accurately. To find the most accurate measures for these and other body parts, we can turn to the work of *anthropometrists*, scientists who make comparative measurements of the human body. Orthodontists, dentists, and plastic surgeons routinely make use of anthropometry to plan for and measure the results of long-term treatment for facial and dental reconstruction. Descriptions of and standards for measurement for the human body are available from sources such as Jones (1997) and Shprintzen (1997).

HEALTH ASSESSMENT

The health care professional directly responsible for health assessment is, of course, a physician. Although diagnosing disease processes is not the speech-language pathologist's primary concern, it *is* our concern to recognize and refer patients who may be experiencing signs of disease. Using visual observation, we can learn to recognize problems such as otitis media, dental caries, chronic allergic reactions, malocclusion, and other medical conditions commonly found in patients with craniofacial anomalies. Recognition of health problems should be followed by referral to the appropriate medical professional, whether or not the patient experiences communication problems resulting from the disease.

IDENTIFYING GENETIC PROBLEMS

As a speech-language pathologist learns to make more discrete patient observations, he or she may notice that those observations fall into a unique pattern or group of symptoms suggestive of a genetically caused problem or syndrome. In ideal professional settings, findings can be presented to members of a diagnostic team for confirmation, assistance, and long-term planning. If team consultation is unavailable locally, findings can be documented and appropriate referrals can be made. Detailed written descriptions of a patient's phenotype, accompanied by explanations of reasons for concern, can appropriately accompany such referrals. Although advanced genetic testing may be required to confirm the presence of genetic problems, obtaining an initial phenotypic description is a first step in this process.

Reassessment and Treatment

The appearance of the craniofacial complex changes over time. For most people, these changes occur naturally as part of the normal growth, development, and aging process. For others, changes may result from disease or trauma. Still other craniofacial changes may be deliberately planned in order to correct or prevent craniofacial abnormalities, or to perfect a less than desirable physical appearance. Because changes brought about by orthodontic treatment or plastic surgery can affect the acquisition, development, and production of normal speech and language, speech pathologists need to monitor these changes carefully. In such cases, systematic documentation of observations is necessary if longitudinal changes in communication development are to be successfully addressed.

Long-Term Treatment Plans and Research

Speech-pathology students sometimes recoil from the idea of conducting research. Such students often express their career goal as a general desire "to help people" by providing speech and language therapy and family counseling. "Research," as these students define it, means a mysterious and difficult set of tasks, most of which are performed in a medical laboratory and none of which directly benefit the patient. Although formal medical research is conducted under stringent laboratory conditions, this is not necessarily the norm for all research projects.

All clinicians conduct research while collecting and recording information about their patients. Most clinicians want to know as much as possible about their patients' communication disorders before beginning treatment. To do that, many clinicians review professional literature to learn current information about specific disorders. This, too, is a step in the research process. Clinicians who compare their own clinical observations to those reported in professional literature have taken an important initial step in planning a formal research study, and some choose to take the process further by defining a problem, systematically collecting data, and analyzing the patterns of information that occur. The final step in the research process occurs when those patterns are analyzed and formally reported, perhaps in a research forum or poster session at a professional meeting. Whenever clinicians present research findings publicly, others have the opportunity to gain understanding about a particular topic and to compare their experiences with colleagues. Ultimately those experiences help all clinicians prepare accurate treatment plans for similar patients. Successful treatment of craniofacial anomalies and their resulting communication problems depends on the development of an accurate knowledge base. As clinicians we have an opportunity to make a difference in the quality of service provided by our profession by engaging in research in our daily environment.

HOW ARE CLINICAL OBSERVATIONS PERFORMED?

Becoming a skilled observer requires knowledge of what to look for and of how to look for it. It also requires practice in applying observational techniques and an anatomical knowledge base for understanding one's observations.

Comprehensive craniofacial evaluations performed by craniofacial teams usually employ several observational methods, including instrumentational assessment, indirect observation, and direct visual observation.

Instrumentational Observation

Observing craniofacial structure and function via specialized techniques such as nasoendoscopy, videofluoroscopy, and computer imaging has become commonplace in major medical centers. Using such instruments, clinicians can observe and measure structures invisible to the unaided human eye and can study complex patterns of muscle movements from multiple vantage points. Instrumentational observation is the technique of choice for observing human chromosomes, viewing and measuring facial bones, photographing the tympanic membrane, and for videotaping the process of velopharyngeal closure during speech production. Instrumentational observation provides examiners with objective, measurable, accurate information about craniofacial structure and function. Data obtained via instrumentational observation is often used for planning orthodontic care and reconstructive surgery. Because instrumentational observation is an expensive, sometimes invasive process, it is most often available in medical settings.

Indirect Visual Observation

Indirect visual observation occurs when clinicians obtain information about a patient's appearance and behavior from sources other than the patient. Examples of this widely available, inexpensive method of observation include descriptive reports written by trained observers (such as dentists or plastic surgeons) and interviews with untrained observers (such as family members). Because indirect visual observations may reflect the observers' biases, we must interpret these observations cautiously. Untrained observers, for example, often describe a patient's appearance in terms of society's standards for beauty or sexual attractiveness. Interestingly, beautiful or sexually desirable features can also be craniofacial anomalies. Notice how two different observers describe a patient with Waardenburg's syndrome:

Untrained Observer (family member): "Ann's appearance is striking. She has beautiful, wide-set, unusually bright-blue eyes. Her hair is very attractive. It's jet black with a streak of white in it just above her forehead. Her boyfriend thinks that white streak makes her look sexy, like a rock star. Her nose is not her best feature. It's pointed, with small nostrils. Her lips are very full and pouty looking. We call them 'Jackson lips'. Her mother, and most of the women in the Jackson family, have mouths like that. I wouldn't describe Ann as beautiful, but she is unique."

Trained observer (speech pathologist): "Ann has dark blue eyes, dark black hair with a white forelock, broad nasal bridge, beaklike nose with small nares, and a mouth with rather full lips. Her facial features resemble those of her biological mother, who accompanied Ann to the diagnostic session. Ann's facial appearance is suggestive of Waardenburg's syndrome. Because hearing loss is a component of that syndrome, I recommend that Ann receive a complete audiological evaluation."

Because indirect observations may vary in accuracy, detail, and thoroughness, they are most useful when supplemented with direct visual observations by trained observers.

Direct Visual Observation

Direct visual observation requires no technology and is cost-effective, noninvasive, and relatively well tolerated by patients. It is a learned skill, requiring time, an anatomical knowledge base, and the ability to make logical conclusions.

Direct visual observation is an essential component of the diagnostic process and as such may be the first element of a complex treatment plan. It is especially useful in diagnostic situations such as large public school screenings, when individual diagnostic time is short and sophisticated diagnostic materials are unavailable. Commercially available oral-facial protocols can provide a starting point for conducting direct visual observations, although they have limitations. These limitations exist in part because no single profile could contain all-inclusive information for every patient and in part because speech pathologists in general are not routinely trained to look beyond the oral-peripheral area for problems that contribute to communication disorders. A variety of protocols and oral-facial examination forms are available for routine evaluations (Dworkin & Culatta, 1980; Mason & Simon, 1977; Shipley & McAfee, 1992; St. Louis & Ruscello, 1981) and for special populations (Coston et al. 1992; Middleton & Pannbacker, 1997; Shipley & McAfee 1992). Additionally, hospitals, clinics, and other work settings often have in-house oral-facial assessment protocols. The majority of currently available general oral-facial protocols designed for routine use by speech-language pathologists and audiologists:

- are designed for general application, rather than specific age or ethnic groups

- have few in-depth guidelines for eye, hair, hand, or skin assessment

- assume the examiner has the expertise to collect accurate, objective data

- assume the examiner understands the *significance* of observations

The remainder of this chapter provides protocols for visually observing diagnostically significant features that are not routinely assessed by commercially available assessment instruments. The diagnostic significance of these observations will be discussed in depth in Chapter 4. Observation of intraoral structures will be discussed here only when the observation provides a new perspective on traditional intraoral diagnostic assessment methods. Use this material to *enhance*, not replace, the traditional intraoral examination.

PROTOCOL FOR DIRECT VISUAL OBSERVATION

As speech pathologists and audiologists, our major interest is in observing a patient's craniofacial appearance. We must remember, however, that the human body functions as a unit. Body parts distant from the head and neck can contribute to the occurrence of communication problems. Begin by observing three basic relationships that apply to the body as a whole and to the craniofacial complex in particular: *size, proportion,* and *symmetry.*

Size

In humans, size is measured in terms of body height and weight. Height and weight measurements reflect an individual's nutritional intake, metabolism, airway structure and function, and genetic background.

Children who receive routine medical care almost certainly have size and weight information recorded in their medical records because pediatricians routinely use growth and development curves to monitor their patients. Individuals who fall in the upper or lower 2% of growth curves are considered abnormally tall or short, overweight or underweight. If growth and development records are unavailable, it is perfectly proper to weigh and measure a patient to obtain these measures. Select growth curves appropriate for the population you are measuring because racial and ethnic variations in normal growth and development do exist.

Obese children may be overweight for a variety of reasons, not all of which have relevance to craniofacial problems. There are approximately a dozen syndromes in which obesity is a feature. Remember, however, that weight gain may be influenced by an individual's level of physical activity, whether or not the individual has a syndrome. In any case, notice individuals who are significantly overweight and use this information in the broader context of other diagnostically significant features.

Problems with linear growth (height) are often associated with multiple anomaly syndromes, many of which have communication disorders and craniofacial anomalies as features. Linear growth is regulated by the *pituitary gland*. The pituitary gland is located deep within the cranial base in the hypophysial fossa of the sphenoid bone. The fossa is visible in lateral cephalograms as the *sella turcica*, an important landmark for craniofacial measurements. The pituitary gland secretes a growth hormone while a baby is in deep sleep state. Damage to the pituitary gland, anomalies of the pituitary gland, or anomalies that have sleep disorders as a component have the potential to affect linear growth. Because pituitary abnormalities are commonly found in patients with brain anomalies, midline abnormalities, and cleft palates, linear growth should be carefully monitored in such patients.

The large doses of radiation sometimes used to control malignant tumors of the head and neck can also cause pituitary problems with resulting deficiency in linear growth. Retinoblastoma, for example, is a malignant ocular neoplasm usually occurring in children under the age of three. Radiation treatment for retinoblastoma sometimes destroys the pituitary gland, resulting in unilateral or bilateral growth deficiency to the face or to the body in general.

Children with sleep apnea sometimes have a reduction in linear growth because they seldom enter a deep sleep state, and therefore the pituitary gland has little time to excrete the growth hormone necessary to achieve normal linear growth (Goldstein et al., 1985). Because patients are seldom observed during a sleep state, caregivers should be asked about a child's sleep habits, especially when disorders of linear growth are suspected.

Proportion

When we observe a patient's body proportions, we want to know that each body part is properly located and that it occupies the amount of space it should occupy *in relation to the rest of the body*. Standards for normal proportions change as a child attains adulthood. Eyes, for example, are proportionally large in the small face of a baby. This is a normal proportional relationship for infants and very young children, but not for adults.

Sometimes the appearance of surrounding body structures tricks our eyes into believing that a particular body part is disproportionate. Very obese individuals, for example, may appear to have proportionally small hands and feet. Because small hands and feet are characteristic features of more than 30 syndromes, it is important to determine if the disproportion between body parts is visual (as in the obese person with normal size hands), or actual (as in a syndrome). In such cases, we can use anthropometric measures of height, weight, and hand and foot size to determine whether true body disproportion actually exists.

Facial Proportions

Standards for normal adult facial proportions are illustrated in Figure 3–1. Notice that the face can be divided into approximately three equal areas: the forehead, midface, and lower face (Figure 3–1A). The distance between the inner canthi (corners) of the eyes (Figure 3–1B) approximately equals that of the alar nasal base width. *Alar* means "wings," in this case the winglike appearance of lateral aspect of the nose. The individual's mouth should be as wide as the distance from the right to left medial limbus (Figure 3–1C). A *limbus* is a border, in this instance, the border between the cornea and the sclera of the eyeball. *Medial* means "middle," or "center," in this case, toward the nose. Observe the location of the lines carefully. Practice observing facial proportions until you can see them without consulting illustrations.

Profile Proportions

Facial proportions can also be observed in profile. Enlow (1990) described a method of profile assessment that can readily be used in any observational situation. Enlow suggested that the clinician imagine a line extending from the center of the patient's orbit looking straight forward. Next, the clinician should imagine a vertical line perpendicular to the orbital line that extends along the surface of the upper lip. Figure 3–2 illustrates the profile of four patients, with Enlow's suggested lines superimposed over their photographs. In each instance, notice the relationship of the chin to the perpendicular line. This relationship is the decisive factor in determining which type of profile a given patient may have. There are three basic profile types: orthognathic, retrognathic, and prognathic. *Gnathic* comes from the Greek word *gnathos*, meaning "jaw."

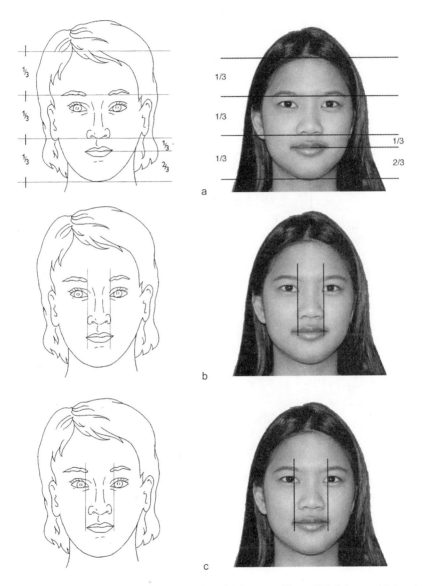

Figure 3–1. Normal facial proportions for adult humans. (From *Cleft Palate and Related Disorders* (p. 145), by G. F. Middleton and M. Pannbacker, 1997, Bisbee, AZ: Imaginart International, Inc. Reprinted with permission. 800–828-1376. Photography by Alice Kahn.)

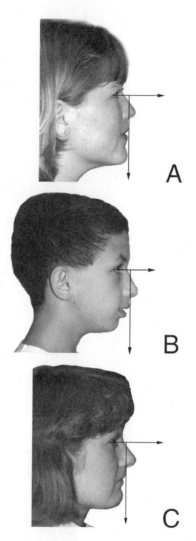

Figure 3–2. Enlow's method of profile assessment: **A.** Orthognathic profile. **B.** Retrognathic profile in a boy with Waardenburg's syndrome. **C.** Slightly retrognathic profile in a normal Caucasian female.

Orthognathic Profile

Ortho means "straight" or "correct." Individuals with an orthognathic profile (Figure 3–2A) have what is considered a good, or socially desirable, profile. Notice that the patient's upper lip and chin just contact the perpendicular line.

Retrognathic Profile

Retro means "backward" or "behind." Individuals with a retrognathic profile have what is commonly called a receding chin. Notice that the patient's chin and lower lip are significantly retruded and that the entire profile has a convex appearance. Retrognathic profile is diagnostically significant because hearing loss often accompanies this profile type, as it does in the boy pictured in Figure 3–2B.

A slightly retrognathic profile (Figure 3–2C) is one that is considered normal and that often occurs in Caucasians. Notice that the upper lip contacts the perpendicular line, while the chin is very slightly retruded.

Prognathic Profile

Pro means "before" or "forward." Individuals with a prognathic profile have a jutting chin, and a tendency to have Class III malocclusion. In profile the entire face has a slightly concave appearance when viewed in profile.

Practice observing proportional relationships on yourself and friends by completing the observational exercises at the end of this chapter. Practice until you gain enough experience in recognizing facial proportions and profile type without consulting illustrations. Remember that each person has two profiles and that two different profile appearances can exist in the same individual. This brings us to the subject of symmetry.

Symmetry

Human beings are bilaterally symmetrical creatures. Most of our body parts are located to the right and left of the spinal column, and most paired body structures are approximately identical in size and shape. Many normal individuals have slightly asymmetrical body parts, but this normal asymmetry is usually not visually distracting.

Facial Symmetry

The right and left sides of the face should be approximately the same size and shape. Bilateral structures (eyes, nares, ears, and both sides of the mouth) should be located on the same plane and should also be approximately the same size and shape. Mobility of moveable bilateral structures (faucial pillars, velum, eyes, eyelids) should be bilaterally symmetrical. Marked unilateral deviation from the midline in mobile bilateral craniofacial structures often indicates cranial nerve pathology. Contrast the slight facial asymmetry of the normal young adult female

(Figure 3–3A) with the more noticeable facial asymmetry of the male with Waardenburg's syndrome (Figure 3–3B.)

Significant facial asymmetry may be caused by syndromes, in-utero deformation, trauma, plastic surgery, or long-term disease processes. Although not everyone with significantly asymmetric body parts is at risk for communication problems, syndromes such as Oculo-Auriculo-Vertebral Spectrum have both communication problems and significant facial asymmetry as major features.

We can also assess size, proportion, and symmetry of individual body parts, particularly those of the craniofacial complex. It is best to observe body parts systematically by selecting vantage points from which to view these structures.

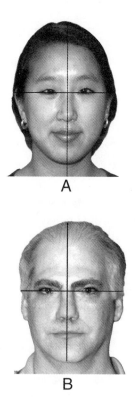

Figure 3–3. A. Slight facial asymmetry in a normal female. **B.** Noticeable facial asymmetry in a male with Waardenburg's syndrome.

Vantage Points

Selecting and using consistent vantage points makes the observational process easier. Basic vantage points include the back of the head (posterior view), the top of the head (superior view), right and left profiles (lateral views), and face to face. Begin by learning how to observe the back of a patient's head.

Posterior Vantage Point

Craniofacially speaking, the posterior vantage point lets the observer view a patient's *hair*, *skin*, and *neck*. Protocols for hair and skin can be used from all vantage points.

**Protocol for Evaluating Hair
From Any Vantage Point**

- Notice *amount* of hair. Observe the entire scalp for areas of sparse or missing hair. Look for signs of traction alopecia in patients who wear tight braids or cornrows.

- Observe *location* of hair relative to neck, forehead, ears, and eyes. In particular, note widow's peak configuration on forehead, eyebrows that meet at midline, flared eyebrows, absent or unusually located sideburns, long or curly eyelashes, and absent lower eyelashes.

- Determine hair *texture*: fine, coarse, brittle, fragile.

- Determine *original* hair *color*. Look for areas of abnormal pigmentation, especially a white forelock in otherwise dark hair. Ask the patient if his or her hair turned gray or silver prematurely, even if the patient's hair is presently dark colored.

- Determine hair *shape*: curly, straight. Ask if hair has been cosmetically curled or straightened.

- Observe hair *growth pattern*. In particular, note the number and location of hair whorls.

Hair provides information about an individual's genetic makeup, in utero development, brain growth, general health, and social preferences. Hair grows from pits in the epidermis called *follicles*. Straight follicles produce straight hair; curly follicles produce wavy or curly hair. Very hairy individuals may have excessive amounts of hair along with an excessive number of hair follicles. This condition is called *hypertrichosis* and must be confirmed by microscopic analysis to determine the number of hair follicles. On the other hand, persons who have excessive body or facial hair in a male pattern (especially women) are said to have *hirsutism*. Hirsute means "shaggy." Although hirsutism may be a normal condition in some ethnic groups, it is also a characteristic feature of more than 20 syndromes (see Appendix). Hirsutism may also result from hormone therapy or from excess production of androgens in some medical disorders.

The congenital absence of hair is called *atrichia*. Atricia commonly occurs in ectodermal dysplasia syndromes, along with congenital absence of teeth and nails. Individuals who have had a normal hair pattern and later lost their hair have a condition called *alopecia*. Alopecia has many possible causes, but is a common inherited condition in adult males. Like hirsutism, alopecia is a characteristic of numerous syndromes (see Appendix), but may also result from chemotherapy, disease processes, dietary conditions, or exposure to teratogens.

Traction alopecia is a type of localized scalp hair loss common among people of African descent. This type of alopecia results from wearing tightly braided hair such as cornrows, weaves, and ponytails. If hair is placed under excessive traction over a long period of time, permanent hair loss may result.

Sometimes midline scalp lesions can be observed in neonates. This condition, *aplasia cutis*, is associated with several syndromes, Adams-Oliver and Johanson-Blizzard syndromes among others. In adults and older children, these lesions may have healed and be visible as bald areas of scar tissue concealed by surrounding hair.

In humans, the *location* of hairlines is influenced by presence and growth of underlying structures such as the vertebrae, the cerebral cortex, the eyes, and the ears. Low posterior hairlines often occur in individuals with short necks. Neck length, in turn, depends on presence and integrity of the cervical vertebrae. Unusual or low posterior hairlines occur frequently in individuals with Down's syndrome (Figure 3–4), fetal alcohol syndrome, and a number of other syndromes that have vertebral anomalies and communication disorders as components.

Forehead hairline is determined in part by the growth of the underlying brain and the position of the eyes. Unusually close- or wide-set eyes are often accompanied by the presence of a central peak of hair extending downward into the forehead (widow's peak). Widow's peak may be a normal variation of forehead hairline or an indication of syndromes such as Aarskog-Scott, Opitz, and Frontonasal Dysplasia Sequence.

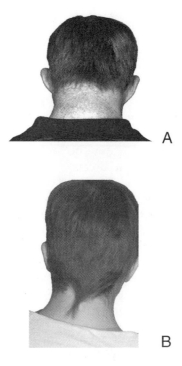

A

B

Figure 3–4. Low posterior hairline (A), and hairline extending far down center of neck (B) in patients with Down's syndrome.

Long, curly, or absent eyelashes are also indicative of specific syndromes (see Appendix). Absence of lower eyelashes is a major characteristic of Treacher Collins syndrome.

Hairline surrounding the ear is dependent on the presence and development of the ear itself. Aberrant hair patterns associated with ear development are usually of two types: the absence of hair where hair should normally occur and the presence of hair where hair should not normally occur. Both conditions are diagnostically significant for presence of syndromes and for hearing loss. Complete absence of the outer ear often results in a lateral area that is devoid of hair, including the hair normally found anterior to the ear (sideburns). Persons with Treacher Collins syndrome and Nager syndrome sometimes have a projection of scalp hair extending into the region of the cheeks.

Texture of normal hair varies widely. The diagnostic significance of very coarse, sparse, brittle, fragile, or fine hair in a given individual must be evaluated against the patient's ethnic background, medical history, and social preferences. Because hair color, texture, and shape can be cosmetically changed, clinicians must be cautious before drawing diagnostic conclusions from visual inspection alone. Be prepared not only to examine hair, but to ask questions about its *original* texture and shape.

It is particularly important to question patients about original hair *color* because prematurely gray hair or a white forelock in otherwise dark hair can be a valuable clue in diagnosing hearing loss. The number of syndromes in which this feature occurs is limited. Waardenburg's syndrome is the most common. Because gray hair is generally considered socially undesirable in a young person, its presence is often concealed with hair dye. Conversely, a white forelock in otherwise dark hair may be perceived as attractive and may be purposely bleached into the hair of a genetically normal person. Very blond, almost silver hair is a characteristic of ectodermal dysplasia syndromes.

A *hair whorl* is an area of hair that spirals outward from a central point. Humans normally have one parietal hair whorl, located several centimeters anterior to the posterior fontanel in infants. Fifty-six percent of single parietal hair whorls are located to the right of the midline; 30% to the left, and 14% are midline (Jones, 1997). The presence of more than one parietal hair whorl in an individual, bilateral hair whorls (Figure 3–5), lack of a parietal hair whorl, and midline or posteriorly located hair whorls are all diagnostically significant because they imply that brain development was anomalous.

The presence of numerous hair whorls, commonly called "cowlicks," in the hairline surrounding the face is also indicative of

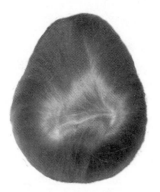

Figure 3–5. Bilateral parietal hair whorls in a 2-year-old boy with developmental disabilities.

anomalous brain growth, as is hair that grows straight upward and backward from the forehead. Aberrant hair growth is a feature of Fetal Alcohol syndrome, Fetal Aminopterin syndrome, and Prader-Willi syndrome, among others.

Observing the posterior vantage point also allows us to observe the patient's skin. Because skin is observable from all vantage points, the observational protocol presented here may be used from any of them.

Protocol for Observing Skin
From Any Vantage Point

- Examine the skin for areas of hyperpigmentation and vitiligo.

- Notice presence and number of café au lait spots.

- Note presence, number, and location of vascular nevi.

- Note presence, number, and location of moles.

- Note additional unusual features such as keloids, hamartomas, or scars.

The study of skin is such a vast topic that an entire medical area (dermatology) is devoted to the treatment of it. Because the appearance of skin provides us with information about an individual's general health, genetic background, and age, clinicians should be prepared to recognize major skin-related features, including normal skin appearance of individuals whose skin color differs from one's own. For a comprehensive overview of skin manifestations in African and Asian individuals, consult Laude et al. (1996). For present purposes, discussion of the skin will be confined to two skin-related issues: pigmentation and nevi (localized overgrowths of melanin forming cells, sometimes called moles). Some pigmentation and nevi-related conditions are components of a broad category of disorders called *hamartoses*. A *hamartoma* is a tumor-like growth that results from faulty tissue organization and development. Communication problems are a component of many hamartoses, including Sturge-Weber syndrome, neurofibromatosis, and LEOPARD syndrome.

All normal skin contains *melanin,* a pigment that darkens on exposure to sunlight. The skin of persons of all races is typically darker on the posterolateral surfaces of the extremities and lighter on the anteromedial surfaces. *Futcher lines* are places where lighter areas meet darker areas;

these are most noticeable in persons with dark skin. Compare the surface of your wrist with the surface of the back of your hand. The skin on your wrist should normally be lighter, no matter what your racial background.

Brown or blue intraoral pigmentation is common in persons of African descent. Seldom apparent at birth, it increases with age, particularly along the gingiva. Intensity of pigmentation correlates with the individual's skin color. Healthy persons of African descent often have increased blue or brown pigmentation on oral mucous membranes and gums, as well as longitudinal pigmented stripes in the fingernails (Laude, 1996). Because abnormal conditions such as lead poisoning, chronic irritation, and melanoma may also produce increased intraoral pigmentation in dark-skinned individuals (Brauner, 1994), it is wise to refer patients to a physician for differential diagnosis.

Abnormal pigmentation in a person of any race is of basically two types: hyperpigmentation and hypopigmentation. Both are more noticeable in dark-skinned persons, and both can be characteristic of syndromes. Although numerous skin pigmentation disorders exist (see Appendix), most are not diagnostically significant for communication disorders. Two, however, do have diagnostic relevance for communication disorders: café au lait spots and vitiligo.

Café au lait spots, as the name suggests, are light coffee-brown hyperpigmented areas, most commonly found on the trunk and near the armpits. They differ from sun-induced pigmentation in that café au lait spots are present in very young infants, are located in places not typically exposed to sunlight, and may cover much larger areas of skin. Café au lait spots are characteristic of a number of syndromes, most notably the numerous types of neurofibromatosis. Six or more such spots measuring 1.5 cm or larger in one individual by 4 years of age is considered diagnostically suggestive of neurofibromatosis (Jones, 1997). The presence of numerous cafe au lait spots in persons of African descent is less diagnostically significant because these spots normally occur more frequently in black children than in other races (Laude et al., 1996).

Vitiligo is an area of depigmented, very white skin that can occur anywhere on the body. Areas of vitiligo appear at birth, or shortly thereafter, and may become larger with age. Vitiligo occurs in persons of all races, but is most noticeable in persons with dark skin. Areas of vitiligo commonly appear on the skin of individuals with Waardenburg's syndrome. Widespread areas of vitiligo may also be characteristic of *piebaldism*, an autosomal-dominant condition common in persons of African descent. Because the characteristics of pibaldism are similar to those of Waardenburg's syndrome, it is impossible to visually distinguish between the two syndromes based on presence of vitiligo alone.

Nevi

A *nevus* can be a localized overgrowth of melanin-forming cells (a mole) or a more serious malformation of the skin with hyperpigmentation and increased vascularity.

Vascular refers to blood supply. Vascularized structures have an abundant and sometimes externally visible blood supply. Vascular nevi can range in appearance from small, strawberry colored areas of skin, to extensive, abnormal, very dark vascularized areas (port-wine stains). Small port-wine stains appear in 40% of all newborns, and persist in 30% of these individuals in adulthood (Wiedemann & Kinze, 1997). Port-wine stains located on the nape of the neck are especially likely to persist into adulthood (Figure 3–6). Port-wine stains occurring in conjunction with other craniofacial anomalies may be useful in diagnosing specific syndromes. In most cases, however, small, isolated port-wine stains are of little diagnostic significance.

Large, usually unilateral port-wine stains that follow the path of the Trigeminal nerve are indicative of Sturge-Weber syndrome; an uncommon disorder with serious central nervous system complications. Seizure disorders frequently accompany this syndrome, as do communication problems related to developmental disabilities.

Other unusual skin features include keloids, scars, and bruises. Although some of these features have implications for issues such as

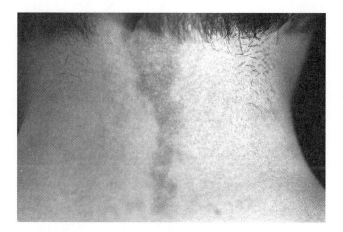

Figure 3–6. A strawberry nevus in a typical location—the nape of the neck. Strawberry nevi are diagnostically significant when they are large, numerous, and occur in conjunction with other anomalies.

child abuse and domestic violence, they are of diagnostic significance for speech pathologists only in that they may be mistaken for craniofacial anomalies.

Keloid tissue, in particular, may be misdiagnosed by novice observers. A *keloid* is a type of scar that forms in some individuals following trauma, burns, or surgical incisions. Keloids may appear as large, firm, benign tissue masses on the skin following even minor events such as ear piercing. Some persons, including persons of African descent, are particularly prone to develop keloid scar tissue. It is easy to mistake keloid scars for preauricular skin tags. For this reason, when observing unusual "growths" in the craniofacial area, it is wise to ask the patient about their origin.

Differential diagnosis of lumps, fibrous lesions, growths and moles is best left to a dermatologist. It is within our purview however, to point out the existence of such growths, especially if the growth is located in an area that is not readily visible (nape of the neck, back of the auricle, intraoral cavity, scalp).

Malignant melanoma (skin cancer) is rare in children and persons of African descent. Regardless of a patient's race or age, however, the presence of any mole with a blue-black color or irregular borders; or a mole that has recently changed in size or shape should always be suspect. Always point out such moles to a patient or the patient's family, and refer the patient to a dermatologist, especially if he or she is fair skinned, has a history of sun exposure, or a history of melanoma in the immediate family.

The presence of numerous skin nevi is diagnostically significant for craniofacial syndromes. The presence of many small moles on the skin is indicative of Waardenburg's syndrome (WS), among others (see Appendix). Because phenotypic expression of WS is quite variable, the presence of many moles in a person whose family is known to have the WS gene may have diagnostic implications.

The neck is the final feature that can be observed from the posterior vantage point.

Protocol for Observing the Neck

- Observe the neck length.

- Observe the skin that covers the neck using previously described protocols.

- Determine if the skin has a normal attachment to the shoulders.

Neck length is related to the presence and structure of the underlying vertebral column. Short necks are usually caused by malformed or missing vertebrae. Noonan's syndrome and Turner's syndrome, among others (see Appendix), have low posterior hairlines and webbed necks as a diagnostic feature. An unusually long neck is a feature of Proteus syndrome, an uncommon type of hamartosis, that also causes abnormal growth of hand, foot, and other bones. Remember that young children may appear to have a large head sitting on top of a long, slender neck. This is a normal relationship, one that changes as the craniofacial complex matures.

Superior Vantage Point

Superior in this instance means observing the top of the patient's head. The superior vantage point lets us observe the patient's hair-growth pattern, fontanels, and skull shape. Evaluate hair-growth pattern using previously described protocols.

Fontanels are the membrane-covered areas between the as yet unjoined skull bones of a newborn infant. Six fontanels are normally present at birth. The size of the anterior and posterior fontanels (Figure 3–7), in particular, is routinely monitored by physicians to be certain the child's development is proceeding properly.

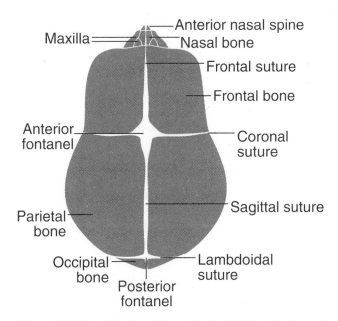

Figure 3–7. Superior view of a newborn's skull, showing fontanels and major cranial bones.

The posterior fontanel is usually no larger than a fingertip in 97% of newborns and should close completely shortly after birth (Jones, 1997). The anterior fontanel closes at about one year and the remainder of the fontanels by 18 months (Enlow, 1982). Too many or too few fontanels may indicate premature or delayed closure of cranial sutures. Unusually large fontanels, or fontanels that do not close on time are also diagnostically significant because they can indicate the presence of congenital hypothyroidism, skeletal dysplasia, intracranial pressure, or certain syndromes (see Appendix).

Protocol for Observing Fontanels

- *Gently* pass your hand over the patient's cranium, noting areas of soft tissue between the harder skull bones. Posterior fontanels should be present only in newborn infants.

- Note the presence of unusually large fontanels in children over 1 year of age.

As brain growth is completed, the bones of the infant's skull grow together and fuse with one another. These lines of fusion are called *sutures*. If a child's brain fails to grow properly, the anterior and posterior fontanels may close prematurely, resulting in a condition called *primary microcephaly*.

In other cases, the rate of brain growth is normal, but the cranial sutures fuse prematurely, a condition called *craniosynostosis*. This premature closure prevents further growth in head circumference, a condition called *secondary microcephaly*. If some cranial sutures close prematurely while others remain open, the brain will continue to grow in the direction of the open sutures, causing the skull to develop an abnormal shape. In both primary and secondary microcephaly, radiographic and CT-scan studies are needed to distinguish between the types of microcephaly. This means that referral is necessary whenever we observe a child with a head size that is smaller than normal or a skull shape that is markedly unusual.

Viewed from above, a skull has a symmetrical shape that may vary according to ethnic background. Symmetrical, oval-shaped skulls are characteristic for normal Caucasians and for many persons of African descent. A more rounded skull shape is normal for Asians.

Protocol for Observing the Skull

- Observe skull shape.
- Observe skull symmetry.

Abnormal skull shape may reflect the growth of the underlying brain or be a result of early closure of cranial sutures. In newborn infants, asymmetrical skull shapes often result from in utero or birth-process deformation. This appearance is often self-correcting. Unusual skull shapes are also indicative of syndromes (See Appendix).

Profile Vantage Point

Profiles, as we have already learned, can offer information about a patient's ethnic background, dental occlusion, and facial development. They also allow the clinician to evaluate hair-growth patterns and external ears bilaterally. Evaluate hair-growth pattern relative to the outer ears using previously described protocols.

Protocol for Evaluating Profiles

- Determine the individual's profile type using Enlow's observational technique.
- Observe size, shape, and symmetry of auricles.
- Notice the size of ear canals.
- Observe the location of outer ears.
- Note auricular and preauricular anomalies.

Humans normally have two ears that, as with all bilateral body parts, should be approximately identical in appearance and placement. Because it is difficult to visualize both ears simultaneously, it helps to make comparative photographs. Figure 3–8 represents a normal ear. Use this photograph as a guide for assessing "normal."

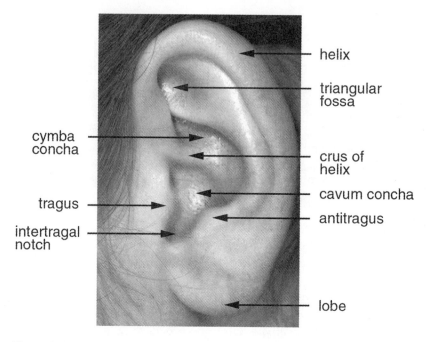

Figure 3–8. Anatomy of a normal human ear.

To evaluate ear *location*, place one end of a straight object (such as a tongue depressor) at the outer canthus of the eye and extend it back toward the posterior part of the head (Figure 3–9). The line thus created should intersect the top third of the ear. It is not uncommon to find marked bilateral ear asymmetry in normal persons (Figure 3–10), as well as in patients with craniofacial syndromes.

The area just anterior to the auricle is called the preauricular area. Small pits (Figure 3–11) or skin tags (Figure 3–12) are often found in this area and may extend downward through the cheek toward the corner of the mouth. Preauricular pits are particularly common in black individuals and are twice as prevalent in females as in males (Jones, 1997). Preauricular skin tags may represent only a minor anomaly or may accompany *microtia* of the ear.

Microtia means absence of the outer ear and is described according to the degree of ear abnormality. If all ear structures are present but smaller than normal, the patient is said to have Grade I microtia. Grade II microtia describes an ear that is malformed externally, one that usually has an external canal ending as a pit. In Grade III microtia, the external ear and ear canal may be absent entirely, and the middle-ear space

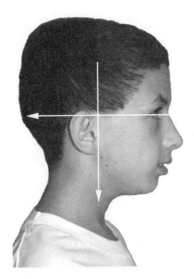

Figure 3–9. Normal ear placement.

and ossicles may also be malformed or reduced in size. All types of microtia can produce conductive hearing losses, with hearing loss being most marked in Grades II and III.

Ears can also protrude from the side of the head. Figure 3–13 shows the location of the auricular muscles that are responsible for holding the ear in its proper location. Congenital absence or hypotonia of one or more of these muscles can result in protruding ear, lop ear (see top photo, Figure 3–10), or protruding-lop ear configurations. Other ear anomalies include incomplete development of the scapha helix, lack of lobules, and lobular creases. Figure 3–14 shows anomalous auricles found in two patients with Down's syndrome. It is important to determine whether an anomaly is congenital or acquired. Always question patients or family members about growths, scars, or pits in the auricular area. Ear lobes especially are frequent sites of keloid scarring following ear piercing. Because individuals with outer-ear anomalies are at risk for conductive hearing loss, they should receive a pure-tone threshold hearing evaluation to rule out this possibility, especially if other craniofacial anomalies are present.

Face-to-Face Vantage Point

Face-to-face is probably the most familiar vantage point to clinicians because it is the view we are accustomed to seeing during intraoral eval-

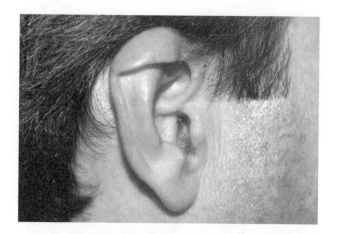

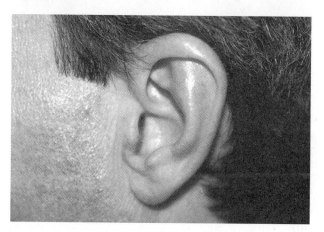

Figure 3–10. Two ears belonging to one normal individual. The ear in the top photo is commonly called a "lop ear" and results from a missing or hypotonic superior auricular ear muscle.

uations. The face-to-face vantage point allows evaluation of skin, eyebrows, and hairline, as well as facial proportion, shape, and symmetry. We can also observe the eyes, nose, mouth, and chin.

Full Face

Use previously described protocols for assessing skin and hair-growth pattern from a full-face vantage point. Remember that the patient's age affects proportional relationships of facial features.

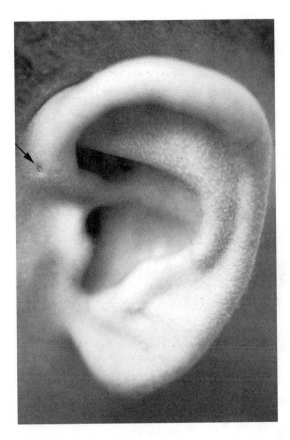

Figure 3–11. Preauricular pits are particularly common in persons of African descent. A pure-tone threshold hearing evaluation should be administered to such patients to rule out presence of hearing loss.

Protocol for Observing the Entire Face

- Evaluate facial proportions and symmetry using previously described protocols.

- Evaluate head size in relation to the rest of the body. Use anthropomorphic measures to evaluate head circumference if necessary.

- Notice the *shape* of the patient's face (triangular, round, square, heart shaped)

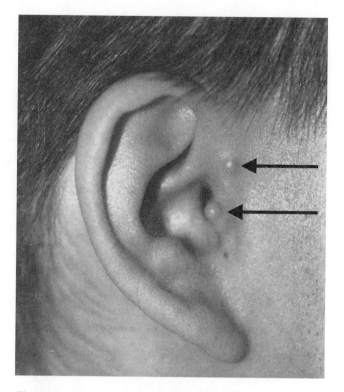

Figure 3–12. Preauricular skin tags or beads of tissue are indications of incomplete auricular formation. This otherwise normal individual also has unusually shaped ear lobes. Hearing evaluations are always a wise precaution in ruling out presence of hearing loss in individuals with ear anomalies.

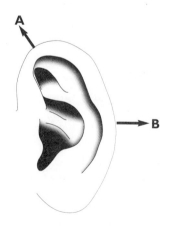

Figure 3–13. The superior auricular muscle (**A**) and the posterior auricular muscle (**B**) help hold the auricle in proper position against the head. Absence or hypotonia of these muscles can produce a variety of anomalies in ear position.

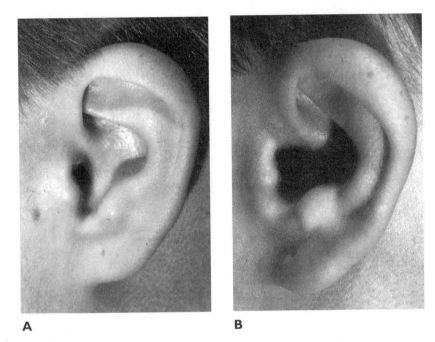

A   **B**

Figure 3–14. Two aberrant ear shapes in persons with Down's syndrome.

After observing the face as a unit, evaluate individual facial features: eyes, nose, lips, and chin.

Eyes

The clinician who is deceived by optical illusions can easily make mistakes while assessing eye orientation, symmetry, and location. The following protocol is helpful, but anthropomorphic measurements may be required for accurate observation of eyes. Figure 3–15 illustrates the appearance of a normal eye and its components. Use this figure as a guide while learning the following protocol.

Protocol for Observing Eyes

- Observe eye *orientation* in the following way: Imagine that a line extends through the *palpebral fissure* (the space between the eyelids) connecting the inner and outer canthi of the right eye. The

(continued)

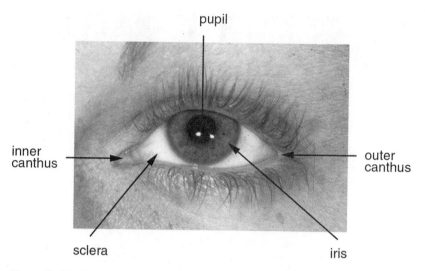

pupil

inner
canthus

outer
canthus

sclera

iris

Figure 3–15. Anatomy of a normal human eye.

line should be horizontal and parallel to the ground regardless of the individual's racial background. Repeat the process for the left eye. Eyes that have an upslanting or downslanting appearance when measured in this way, have an abnormal orientation.

- Extend the imaginary line to connect the inner and outer canthi of both eyes (Figure 3–16). If the imaginary line is horizontal and parallel to the ground, the eyes are placed symmetrically in the face. Upward- or downward-sloping lines indicate asymmetric eye placement.

- Notice eye *position* (distance of the eyes from each other).

- Observe that both eyes and all their components are *present* and are of the same size.

- Look for the presence of cataracts.

- Examine the pupil of the eye; it should be centrally located.

- With the patient looking straight forward, shine a penlight flashlight toward the bridge of the patient's nose. Notice the symmetry of the reflections of the penlight in the patient's eyes. Patients with normal eye *convergence* (ability of both eyes to converge on the object they are viewing) will have bilateral, symmetrical light reflections from the eyes. Patients with problems of convergence have *strabismus*. If one light reflection turns outward toward the side of the face, the patient has *exotropia*. If one light reflection turns inward toward the nose, the patient has *esotropia*.

- Observe the color of the sclera; it should be white.
- Notice the appearance of the iris, its color, and its relationship to the pupil.
- Observe the eyelids for clefts.
- Observe the eyelashes.
- Note the presence of epicanthal folds.

Human beings normally have two eyes that should be the same size. *Anophthalmia* (absence of an eye) or bilateral *microphthalmia* (small eyes) are frequent components of syndromes (see Appendix). Because it is difficult to make accurate visual assessments of eye size, clinicians must use the length of the palpebral fissure as a reflection of eye size. Use a rigid ruler to make this and other eye measurements, and then compare them to anthropomorphic standards. A short palpebral fissure length indicates microphthalmia. Refer such patients to an ophthalmol-

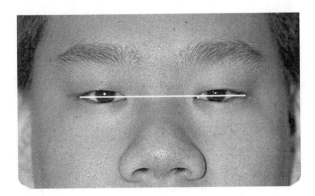

Figure 3–16. Normal eye orientation. Contrary to popular belief, normal eyes of Asian individuals have a horizontal, not slanted, location on the face. Epicanthal folds may deceive the observer by by obscuring the inner canthi and creating the visual suggestion of slanted eyes.

ogist, particularly if other facial anomalies are present or if the patient shows signs of visual impairment.

Normal-sized eyes may appear large if they are bulging from their sockets. The presence of bulging eyes is called *exorbitism* or *exophthalmus*. Bulging eyes are usually not abnormally large, they simply look large because much of the globe of the eye is visible. A variety of serious conditions may cause bulging eyes, including intracranial pressure, premature closure of cranial sutures, shallow eye orbits, and a variety of conditions such as Crouzon's syndrome and Apert's syndrome (see Appendix).

The *sclera* (covering tissue of the eyeball) is often thin with a blue appearance in individuals with ectodermal dysplasia syndromes. Such syndromes are associated with a number of communication disorders resulting from deafness, cleft palate, and mental retardation. *Ectoderm* is an embryonic tissue that forms the covering tissues of many anatomical structures. Individuals whose eyes have blue schlera may also have hypoplastic fingernails, digital anomalies, microtia of auricles, absent eyelashes, sparse hair, and thin or absent tooth enamel. Hair and eyes are often light colored, and hair may be wiry or brittle. Teeth are often missing (*anodontia*) or cone shaped, and cleft lip, cleft palate, or both are sometimes present. Examine the appearance of all covering structures (hair, skin, eyelashes, fingernails), when ectodermal dysplasia is suspected.

Eye color can be an important diagnostic clue for the presence or future development of hearing loss in humans or animals. Cat and dog fanciers know that odd-eyed (one blue eye, one eye of another color) or blue-eyed white dogs or cats are likely to be deaf. Human beings with Waardenburg's syndrome (WS) often experience similar anomalies. WS is carried as an autosomal dominant genetic trait, and its symptoms include (among other things) bright-blue eyes, heterochromia iridium, hearing loss, epicanthal folds, and pigmentation disorders. Figure 3–17 shows the variable expression of phenotypic expression in family members with Type 1 and Type 2 WS. Patients who have the WS gene are at risk for developing hearing loss throughout their lifetime, with variable time of onset. Such patients should receive routine hearing testing throughout their lifetime, especially during childhood while speech and language are developing. The presence of heterochromia iridium in any patient calls for further investigation into the patient's genetic background and for a thorough audiological evaluation. Other syndromes that have anomalous or unusual eye color and patterns associated with them are listed in the Appendix.

When clinicians observe eye *position*, they want to know if the eyes are located the proper distance from one another. Eyes may be (or appear to be) too close together or too far apart. It is fairly easy to make a preliminary assessment about eye position by taking three additional

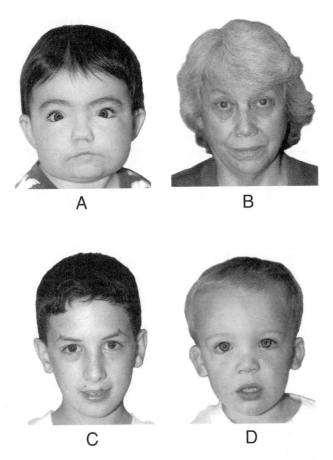

Figure 3–17. Variable phenotypic expression in four individuals with Waardenburg's syndrome. Infant (A) has Waardenburg's type I with unusual facial features and bright-blue eyes; adult (B) has Waardenburg's type 2 with blue eyes and normal hearing; her grandson (C) has Waardenburg's type 2 with a unilateral hearing loss; infant (D) has Waardenburg's type I with profound hearing loss, which is being treated by a cochlear implant.

eye measurements: inner canthal distance, interpupillary distance, and outer canthal distance (Figure 3–18). If the orbits (the bony framework) of the eyes are truly set far apart in the face, the individual is said to have *orbital hypertelorism*. All three of the above measures must be increased in order for hypertelorism to exist.

Patients with closely set eyes, or *hypotelorism*, have a reduced intercanthal, interpupillary, and outer canthal distance. Both hypertelorism and hypotelorism may occur as an isolated feature or as part of a syndrome.

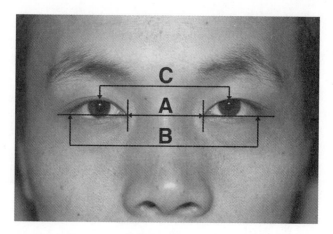

Figure 3–18. Eye measurements. Inner canthal distance (A), outer canthal distance (B), and interpupillary distance (C).

Epicanthal folds occur when nasal bridge bones are flattened or hypoplastic. Epicanthal folds occur frequently in babies and young children, particularly Asian and African children, before facial bone growth is complete. Epicanthal folds remain a normal feature of adult Asian faces, and slight epicanthal folds may be a normal feature of adult Caucasians (Figure 3–19).

Sometimes individuals have epicanthal folds that obscure the inner canthi of the eyes (Figure 3–20). In this case, the outer canthal and interpupillary distances are often within normal limits, but the inner canthal measurements are increased. This condition is called *dystopia canthorum* or *telecanthus*. Dystopia canthorum gives the patient a "cross-eyed" look and may deceive an observer into making an incorrect diagnosis of *strabismus*.

True strabismus, the inability of the eyes to focus together on an object, may occur if the muscles responsible for eye mobility are abnormal in structure or if the cranial nerves supplying those muscles are missing or damaged. Cranial nerve or muscle anomalies may also produce *esotropia*, one eye turning inward toward the nose; *exotropia*, one eye turning outward; and *amblyopia*, eyes that wander from the desired visual target. Central nervous system lesions may produce *nystagmus*, rapid, side-to-side movements of the eyeballs. Apart from the fact that these conditions are often found in syndromes featuring communication disorders, these problems impair the patient's vision. Such patients should always be referred to an ophthalmologist for corrective treatment.

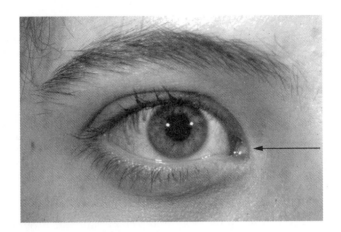

Figure 3–19. Slight epicanthal fold in a normal Caucasian individual. Such folds are often present in normal persons with low nasal bridges.

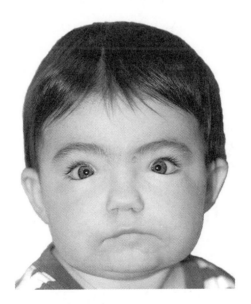

Figure 3–20. Dystopia canthorum in an infant with Waardenburg's syndrome. Also note eyebrow configuration, wide, flat nasal bridge, and bright-blue eyes.

Aniridia means a missing iris. The entire iris or only a portion of it may be absent giving the iris a keyhole appearance. This condition is called *coloboma* iridis and may indicate an underlying problem with the retina, the optic nerve, or both. Retina and optic nerve assessment requires special training and equipment; patients with coloboma iridis should be referred to an ophthalmologist. Colobomas of the retina and optic nerve are indicators of serious problems, such as holoprosencephaly (see Appendix).

Eyelashes should be present on top and bottom eyelids. Notice presence of unusually long, thick, or curly lashes on the upper lid. Be sure the lids themselves are mobile and that they have no notches in them.

Not all eye anomalies are syndrome related, nor do they always suggest the presence of communication disorders. The patient in Figure 3–21 has heterochromia; in this case, one blue eye and one brown eye. A closer look at the blue eye (left eye in photograph) reveals scar tissue on the surface of the iris and pupil. This patient is legally blind in this eye as a result of an eye injury received when his suspender strap hit him in the eye during infancy. Always ask the patient or the patient's caregiver how and when eye anomalies were acquired. Eye-color changes associated with Waardenburg's syndrome, for example, may occur at any time during the patient's lifetime.

Nose

The nose, like hair, is a site of frequent cosmetic change. Ask the patient about previous nasal trauma or cosmetic surgery.

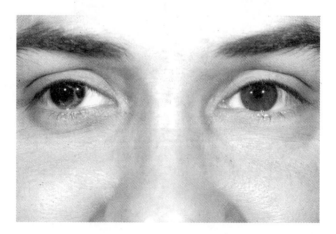

Figure 3–21. Eye trauma, resulting in loss of brown pigmentation and scar tissue on iris of eye (left). Eye on right is normal.

Protocol for Observing the Nose

- Look at the appearance of the nose in profile.

- Notice the size and symmetry of the nose relative to the patient's gender, age, and race.

- Observe size and symmetry of the *nares* (nasal openings).

Evaluate the appearance of the nose for symmetry using previously described protocols. The nasal septum is made of cartilage, a flexible tissue that is subject to mechanical deformation. Individuals with a history of allergies or sinus problems frequently have asymmetrical noses resulting from a lifelong habit of nose rubbing, blowing, and wiping.

Although there are always exceptions, Caucasian individuals are likely to have longer, thinner noses than persons of African and Asian descent. Persons of African descent in particular are likely to have a broad nasal bridge, with wide, flaring nostrils.

Patients with midface deficiencies may have unusual nasal configurations, as may patients who were born with cleft lip, cleft palate, or a combination of the two. Although many people have one nostril that is larger than the other, significant asymmetry of the nares may indicate a history of trauma, a deviated septum, or nasal obstruction. Listen carefully to the speech and resonance characteristics of such patients, and observe the person's face for signs of facial grimacing during conversational speech. Listen for nasal rustle during quiet breathing.

Mouth

The mouth is formed by the fusion of bilateral first arch structures. Use Figure 3–22 as a guide for the appearance of normal circumoral structures.

Protocol for Observing Mouth and Lips

- Ask the patient to close the lips and keep them together in a relaxed position. Observe the relative *width of the mouth* from each corner to the center of the lips. Notice if one side of the mouth seems wider than the other.

- To assess facial or mandibular *symmetry*, ask the patient to hold a tongue depressor horizontally between the teeth, flat side down, from right to left. As the patient faces you with the head upright, the tongue depressor should be parallel with the ground. If the tongue depressor rests at an angle while the patient's head is upright, facial or mandibular asymmetry may be present.

- Observe the lower lips for signs of pits that may or may not have a mucus-like discharge.

- Observe the shape of the mouth as a whole.

- Observe the shape of the lips at rest and as the patient smiles.

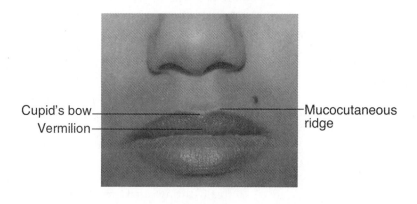

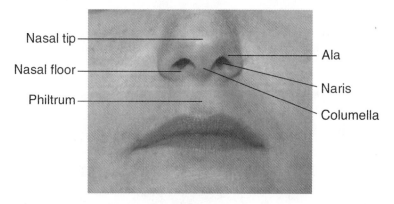

Figure 3–22. Normal circumoral structures of mouth (A) and nasal area (B).

Lips should be symmetrical in structure and in function. Symmetrical function of the facial nerve VII and the lip musculature is usually assessed during the oral-peripheral examination by asking the patient to smile and pucker the lips while the examiner notes lip mobility and symmetry.

Unusually wide or narrow mouth openings may be present unilaterally or bilaterally. *Macrostomia* (abnormally wide mouth) and *microstomia* (abnormally small mouth) results when too much or too little fusion occurs between the maxillary and mandibular processes of the embryonic face. These conditions are present in a number of craniofacial syndromes in which communication disorders are present (see Appendix).

Look at the lower lips carefully and notice the presence of small pits. These may or may not contain a mucus-like substance. Such pits are an indication of Van der Woude's syndrome, a hereditary condition that often has cleft lip as another feature.

Be particularly aware of a mouth that is triangular in shape, with prominent downturned corners of the lips. Full lips, downturned corners of the mouth, and prominent "cupid's bow" outline of the upper lips are indicative of conditions such as Robinow's syndrome, Russell-Silver syndrome, and Duplication 9p syndrome, all of which have facial anomalies and communication disorders as components.

The presence of a deep central dimple in the chin may suggest insufficient fusion of the right and left mandibular processes at midline. In most cases, this lack of fusion is restricted to soft tissues, but occasionally the problem includes mandibular midline anomalies.

Additional Diagnostically Significant Features: Hands

After observing craniofacial features from the aforementioned vantage points, complete the observational process by observing the patient's hands. Although hands are not part of the craniofacial complex, they are symmetrical structures that can provide differential diagnostic clues between disease processes, trauma, and syndromes. Figure 3–23 shows the anatomy of a normal hand. Use this figure as a guide when making observations.

Protocol for Observing Hands

- Notice size and symmetry of hands.
- Measure length of digits relative to the palms; compare to anthropomorphic standards.

(continued)

- Notice structure of digits.

- Count the number of digits.

- Observe dermatoglyphic patterns of palms and fingertips.

- Observe presence, color, and structure of fingernails.

As previously mentioned, hands may be abnormally large or small (or they may appear to be so because of the patient's overall height and weight). Use anthropomorphic measures to make absolute judgments of hand size. Measure palmar length by placing a ruler on the flexion creases at the wrist and the base of the middle finger. Also measure from the flexion crease at the base of the middle finger to the finger tip, not including the overlying fingernail. Compare these measures to anthropomorphic standards.

External structure of the hand can be observed directly and the internal structure of the finger bones (*phalanges*) indirectly. Normal hands have five straight digits (four fingers and a thumb) separated by spaces. Normal digits are intersected at intervals by *flexion creases* overlying the finger joints and marking the borders of the phalanges. *Phalanx* means "a company of soldiers." Each hand should have a total of 14 phalanges, three in each finger and two in each thumb. All phalanges should be approximately the same length. For observational purposes, assume that the length of the phalanges is equivalent to the length of space between the flexion creases. *Distal* phalanges are located at the tips of the fingers, *proximal* phalanges are adjacent to the palm of the hand, and phalanges located between the proximal and distal phalanges are *middle* phalanges. Thumbs have no middle phalanges. The size and shape of the fingernails approximates the appearance of the underlying distal phalanges.

Digital anomalies include extra digits, absent digits, extra phalanges, absent phalanges, and inward deviation of phalanges (*clinodactyly*). Clinodactyly and *camptodactyly* (curved fingers caused by flexion contracture of the interphalangeal joint) are common anomalies of the little finger, both in normal individuals and in individuals with syndromes.

Congenital absence of the hand or forearm may be a feature of a syndrome, or the result of exposure to in utero teratogens such as thalidomide. *Syndactyly* is a condition in which fingers are fused to one another. If the fingers are joined by skin only, the condition is *simple syn-*

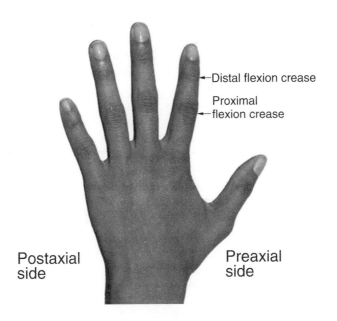

Distal flexion crease

Proximal
flexion crease

Postaxial
side

Preaxial
side

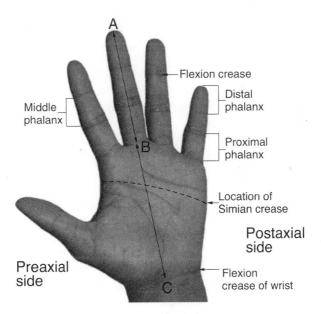

A

Flexion crease

Distal
phalanx

Middle
phalanx

B

Proximal
phalanx

Location of
Simian crease

Postaxial
side

Preaxial
side

C

Flexion
crease of wrist

Figure 3–23. Anatomy of a normal hand showing flexion creases and location of phalanges.

dactyly; complex syndactyly occurs when both skin and bone are joined. Apert's syndrome is associated with *bilateral acrosyndactyly*, a deformity that produces distally joined fingers with a space between the proximal areas of the fingers.

Syndactyly may also result from injuries that have not received proper treatment. If hands are seriously burned, for example, scar tissue may form between digits as the burn heals, fusing the digits together.

Polydactyly (extra digits) is a duplication problem. The problem may be transmitted as a single genetic trait, or it may be associated with life-threatening syndromes. Polydactyly is subclassified into *preaxial* and *postaxial* types. In preaxial polydactyly, the additional digits occur on the thumb side of the hand; in postaxial polydactyly, extra digits occur on the side opposite the thumb. Because preaxial and postaxial polydactyly is sometimes syndrome specific; identifying the type of polydactyly is important for differential diagnosis. Partial rudimentary postaxial polydactyly is also race specific, occurring in 100–300 persons of African descent, or 10 times more frequently than in Caucasians (Wiedemann & Kunze, 1997).

Absent phalanges or extra phalanges are common components of multiple anomaly syndromes. Thumbs that contain an extra phalanx may give the hand a five fingered (*triphalangeal thumb*) appearance. Triphalangeal thumb is diagnostically significant because its presence is associated with syndromes that have sensorineural hearing loss as a component (see Appendix).

Hypoplastic (small) or *aplastic* (absent) fingernails are characteristic of more than two dozen syndromes (see Appendix). Nail splitting, discoloration, and longitudinal ridging are also common symptoms of syndrome-related disorders. Because these symptoms may also indicate disease processes, trauma, or self-inflicted injury, put fingernail appearance in perspective, and use it only to confirm a diagnosis, not *as* diagnosis of the presence of a syndrome.

Blue or dark colored fingernails (*cyanosis*) may indicate heart or lung disorders in Caucasian individuals; however, it is normal for fingernails of persons of African descent to be pigmented and to develop dark, longitudinal ridges with aging.

Anthropomorphic standards for hands and feet are part of an overall body of information called *dermatoglyphics* (skin writing). Dermatoglyphics is the study of the patterns on the skin of the sole of the foot, the palms of the hands, the fingers and the toes. Taking handprints and footprints of newborn babies is standard practice in many hospitals. *Simian* means "monkeylike," and refers to the horizontal crease that appears in a human palm, making it resemble a monkey's palm. Although normal individuals occasionally have simian creases across their palms, the appearance of a simian crease in conjunction with unusual facial features is diagnostic of Down's syndrome. As previously mentioned, newborn babies, particularly those of African descent, may have facial features similar to Down's syndrome. In such instances, dermatoglyphic observation is useful in confirming a suspected diagnosis of conditions such as Down's syndrome.

SUMMARY

Observation of the whole patient can help clinicians determine whether a problem exists, diagnose what that problem is, and recognize other problems that are likely to be present. Diagnostic protocols provide a systematic method of observing patients and collecting data. Information obtained from observations contributes to the overall body of information about specific communication disorders. Collecting information is an initial step in the diagnostic process, one that must be taken before differential diagnosis can begin.

Observation Exercise 1: Observing Facial Proportions

Tools: a good quality mirror, a felt tip pen or lipstick, and a wooden ruler or straight piece of cardboard. Use a good quality mirror; cheap mirrors will distort your reflection.

For best results, comb your hair away from your face, so that the entire hairline is visible. Ask a friend to trace the outline of your face on the mirror with lipstick or a felt tip pen as you stand perfectly still. Using Figure 3–1 as a guide, ask your friend to position the ruler vertically on the mirror so that it intersects the reflection of the inner canthi of your right eye. What is the relationship between the lower part of your nose and the ruler? Repeat for the left eye. Is the distance between the inner canthi of your eyes approximately equal to the width of your alar nasal base?

Let your friend place the ruler horizontally so that it connects the reflection of the right medial limbus of your eye to the reflection of the left medial limbus of your eye. Draw this line with the felt-tip pen or lipstick. Place the ruler horizontally on the reflection of your mouth, measuring from the right to the left corner. Draw a line on the mirror with the felt pen. Compare the width of both lines. They should be approximately equal.

Observation Exercise 2: Observing Facial Symmetry

Ask your friend to measure facial symmetry while you stand perfectly still. Let your friend place the ruler vertically so that it intersects the midpoint of your nasal bridge and the midpoint of your chin. Draw a line on the mirror with the felt-tip pen. Position the ruler horizontally over your reflection so that it intersects both the right and left inner canthi of your eyes. Is one side of your mouth or one of your eyes positioned significantly higher or lower than the other? Smile. Does one side of your mouth move higher than the other? Does a dimple appear when you smile? Unilaterally? Bilaterally? Do you have a mole or birthmark on your face? What other features make your face asymmetrical? Step away from the mirror. What shape is the image drawn on the mirror (oval, round, triangular, square)?

Observation Exercise 3: Observing Profile Type

Sit quietly in a public place and observe the profile types of the people around you. Use Enlow's technique for visualizing profile type and Figure 3–2 as a guide. Practice seeing profiles until you can recognize profile type without referring to the photographs. Try to find five examples of each type of profile. Observe profiles of very young children and of senior citizens. Is one type of profile more common in one group than another? Why might this be so? Observe profiles of people of different races. Is one profile type more common than another?

REFERENCES

Brauner, G. J. (1994). Pigmentation and its disorders in blacks. In N. Levine (Ed.), *Pigmentation and pigmentary disorders* (pp. 439–464). Ann Arbor, MI: CRC Press.

Christianson, A. L, Kromberg, J. G. R., & Viljoen, E. (1995). Clinical features of black African neonates with Down's syndrome. *East African Medical Journal, 72*, 306–310.

Coston, G. N., Sayetta, R. B., Friedman, H. I., Weinrich, M. C., Macera, C. A., Meeks, K., McAndrews, S. K., & Morales, K. S. (1992). Craniofacial screening profile: Quick screening for congenital malformations. *Cleft Palate-Craniofacial Journal, 29*, 87–91.

Dworkin, J., & Culatta, R. (1980). *Dworkin-Culatta oral mechanism examination.* Nicholasville, KY: Edgewood Press, Inc.

Enlow, D. H (1990). *Facial growth* (3rd ed.). Philadelphia: W. B. Saunders Co.

Goldstein, S., Shprintzen, R. J., Wu, R. H. K., Thorpy, M. J., Hahm, S. Y., Marion, R., Sher, A. E., & Saenger, P. (1985). Correction of deficient sleep entrained growth hormone release and obstructive sleep apnea by tracheostomy in achondroplasia, *Birth Defects, 21,* 93–101.

Jones, K. L. (1997). *Smith's recognizable patterns of human malformation* (5th ed.). Philadelphia: W. B. Saunders Co.

Laude, A. L., Kenney, J. A., Prose, N. S., Treadwell, P. A., Resnick, S. D., Gosain, S., & Levy, M. L. (1996). Skin manifestations in individuals of African or Asian descent. *Pediatric Dermatology, 13,* 158–168.

Mason, R., & Simon, C. (1997). An orofacial examination checklist. *Journal of Language Speech Hearing Services in Schools, 8,* 155–164.

Middleton, G. F., & Pannbacker, M. (1997). Speech-language screening and assessment. *In Cleft palate and related disorders* (pp. 113–174). Bisbee, AZ: Imaginart International, Inc.

Shipley, K. G., & McAfee, J. G. (1992). *Assessment in speech-language pathology: a resource manual.* San Diego, CA: Singular Publishing Group.

Shprintzen, R. J. (1997). *Genetics, syndromes, and communication disorders.* San Diego, CA: Singular Publishing Group, Inc.

St. Louis, K., & Ruscello, D. (1981). *The Oral Mechanism Screening Examination.* Baltimore: University Park Press.

Wiedemann, H. R., & Kunze, J. (1997). *Clinical syndromes.* London: Times Mirror International Publishers Limited.

CHAPTER 4

UNDERSTANDING YOUR OBSERVATIONS: DIFFERENTIAL DIAGNOSIS AND PATIENT DISPOSITION

Information collected from direct visual observations must be analyzed and interpreted correctly to develop appropriate treatment plans. In ideal professional settings, differential diagnosis may be conducted by an interdisciplinary team of health care professionals who have results of instrumental observations and the patient's complete medical history to assist in making diagnostic conclusions. Additional diagnostic expertise is often available to team members via Internet listserves, interdisciplinary contacts with professionals at other major medical centers, and craniofacial computer databases. Speech-language pathologists (SLPs) who are members of such teams enjoy a significant advantage over solitary SLPs practicing in public schools or isolated clinical settings.

Does this mean those SLPs who are unaffiliated with major medical centers should automatically refer every patient who appears to have a craniofacial anomaly to the nearest craniofacial team? Not necessarily. Remember that not every characteristic that strays from the norm is an anomaly, not every anomaly is genetic, and not every genetic anomaly has serious implications for craniofacial development or for the development of communication disorders. For these reasons, among others, the ability to make accurate differential diagnoses is a valuable skill for all SLPs. Before referring patients for what may be a lengthy and expensive diagnostic evaluation at a major craniofacial center, SLPs must be reasonably certain that the patient could benefit from such services and that the time and expense of such treatment are warranted. This can be done by making accurate observations, interpreting those observations correctly, understanding the implications of those observations, backing up observations with additional diagnostic testing, and reviewing *all* treatment options. In the previous chapter, protocols for making accurate visual observations of the craniofacial complex were described. This chapter explains how to interpret diagnostic observations, how to understand the implications of those observations, and how to proceed once a preliminary diagnosis has been reached.

DIFFERENTIAL DIAGNOSIS

No matter what the setting, professionals arrive at diagnoses after careful consideration of *all* available data, not just data obtained from direct visual observations. Even in limited diagnostic screenings, SLPs are likely to have basic information about the patient's general health and results of previous medical or psychological testing in addition to information obtained from speech and hearing screenings. Sometimes school nurses, counselors, or classroom teachers can offer additional observations about a child's communication skills. Taken together, these sources can provide a considerable body of information to supplement visual observations.

Obtaining Background Information

Ideally, diagnosticians should have the opportunity to collect case history information prior to the initial diagnostic session. When genetic disorders are suspected, obtaining accurate case information becomes even more critical to the diagnostic process. Clinics and hospitals sometimes obtain initial case history information in advance by mailing generic or specific case history forms to the patient's family. If this information is completed and returned before the patient's appointment, it can be used to narrow the diagnostic focus and to provide direction for the remainder of the assessment process. When genetic disorders are suspected, case history information also can be used to establish modes of inheritance, a phenotypic spectrum, and a natural history of the suspected disorder (Shprintzen, 1997). Obtaining written case history information in advance can work well when families are well educated, literate, and speak English fluently.

The problem for many SLPs, however, is that circumstances may place case history collection at the end of the process, rather than at the beginning. Public health, school, or Head Start screenings often evaluate populations of very young children, many of whom have received inadequate health care. In such groups, initial diagnosis of communication problems and craniofacial anomalies is commonplace. Children who are categorized as at risk for craniofacial anomalies or genetic disorders during initial screenings may be retested or referred for in-depth diagnosis at a university clinic or medical center. During initial screenings, there is little time or opportunity to conduct family or patient interviews nor are family members generally present to provide such information.

SLPs who conduct initial diagnostic screenings, work with populations of functionally illiterate patients, or treat patients who speak English as a second language may have limited access to extensive case history information. In a sense, they must work backward by first collecting diagnostic information and then obtaining background information from medical records or by interviewing family members.

The art of conducting case history interviews is acquired through lifelong practice. Sources for case history protocols for patients with craniofacial anomalies include Emerick and Haynes (1986); Middleton and Pannbacker (1997); Morris and Hall (1994); Peterson and Marquardt (1994); and Shipley & McAfee (1992). (A particularly helpful set of guidelines for obtaining detailed case histories of patients with craniofacial anomalies can be found in Shprintzen's [1997] *Genetics, Syndromes, and Communication Disorders*.) Table 4–1 provides an outline of significant areas to explore during initial interviews with patients suspected of having genetic disorders. By comparing information obtained from case history interviews to visual observations and instrumentational test results, the likelihood of achieving an accurate diagnosis increases.

Table 4–1. Topics to Explore While Taking Case History Information

Family Background

May be asked of any family member:
- What is your family's ethnic background?
- Is there a family history of inheritable conditions such as sickle cell anemia, Tay-Sachs disease, or cystic fibrosis?
- Is there a family history of neurological conditions such as multiple sclerosis, Wilson's disease, Huntington's chorea, cerebral palsy, or spina bifida?
- Is there a family history of cardiovascular disease?
- Do hearing loss or visual problems run in the family?
- Is there a family history of premature, nonaccident-related, death?
- Is there a family history of twinning or multiple births?

Prenatal History

Preferably asked of biological mother (or caregiver who is informed of mother's history):
- Was this your first pregnancy? How many pregnancies have you had?
- Do you have a history of difficult pregnancies, stillbirths, or spontaneous abortions?
- Did you receive fertility treatments to assist conception?
- Did you have sonograms or amniocentesis performed during your pregnancy? What were the results?
- Was this pregnancy unusual? If so, how?
- Did you have an illness or fever during your pregnancy?
- Did you take prescription medication while pregnant? What was it? What was it prescribed for?
- Did you smoke, drink alcohol, or use recreational drugs during this pregnancy?
- What was the length of this pregnancy? Did it last longer than your predicted delivery date? How much longer?
- Was your child delivered earlier than your predicted delivery date? How much earlier?
- Did you receive regular medical attention throughout your pregnancy?
- Where did you deliver your child? In your home? In a hospital?
- Who assisted you in delivering your child? Your doctor? Public health nurse? Midwife? Family member?

Perinatal History

- Was this a multiple birth?
- How long were you in labor?
- Was this a cesarean delivery?
- Did you practice natural childbirth?
- Did you receive local or general anesthesia during delivery?
- Were there complications to the delivery? What were they?
- Was there anything unusual about this delivery?

(continued)

Table 4–1. (continued)

Postnatal History

- How much did your baby weigh? What was his/her length? What were his/her Apgar scores?
- Did you or your baby need special life support measures during or immediately after delivery?
- How soon after birth were you and your baby able to go home?
- Were you able to successfully breast feed or bottle feed your baby?

General Family History

Asked of both biological parents (or of caregivers who are informed about history of biological parents):
- How many children do you have? Are they all living? (If children have died, follow up with specific questions as to time and cause of death.)
- How old were you when your children were born?
- Are any members of your family mentally retarded?
- Does anyone in your family have learning disabilities?
- Does anyone in your family have birth defects or unusual facial features?
- Who does your child most resemble?

Tips for Obtaining Case Histories

- If preliminary case history information is available from prediagnostic questionnaires, remember to orally review this information with the patient. Use this opportunity to probe for missing information or to clarify ambiguous statements.

- Never assume that patients are literate.

- Never assume that patients understand professional vocabulary. Even well-educated patients may misinterpret "simple" professional terms. Unnecessarily stressful situations may arise because of dual meanings for such basic words as *profound*. During one counseling session, for example, a parent who was also a special education teacher was informed that her child had a *"profound unilateral hearing loss."* She interpreted this statement to mean that her child was going to be profoundly mentally

(continued)

retarded and became distraught. Her understanding of *profound* related to intellectual capacity; the audiologist's definition of *profound* related to degree of hearing loss. Carefully explain exactly what you mean when asking questions or reporting diagnostic findings.

- Ask important questions several times in several different ways throughout the interview. Restate questions in several forms, using different words if possible. For example, a recent interview with a patient who was experiencing intermittent aphonia and breathy voice produced no information regarding etiology of these problems. Throughout the interview, the patient was asked the following questions: Have you ever had an injury to your head or neck? Have you ever had surgery to your head or neck? Have you ever had an illness such as arthritis or meningitis or a spinal problem that affected your neck or head? The answer was "no" in all cases. Finally, at the end of the interview, the patient was asked what she did as a hobby. She replied that she enjoyed horseback riding. When asked, "Have you ever had a fall and injured yourself?" she replied, "Why yes, I had a bad fall last summer and broke my right collarbone." When asked why she had not mentioned that fact when she was questioned about head and neck injuries, the patient replied, "Well, you said, *head and neck*, and my collarbone is part of my *shoulder*."

- Realize that interviewees may not always tell the truth or relate all pertinent information during the initial interview. Often guilt or concern over the source of an inherited anomaly may obscure the facts necessary to identify that anomaly. Several interviews may be necessary before the interviewee is ready to reveal information about hereditary conditions.

- Be aware that caregivers or patients may not reveal significant diagnostic information if they believe that illegal or immoral behavior on their part contributed to the problem. Interviewees may be unwilling or unable to confront the consequences of physical abuse, use of illegal "recreational" substances, or ingestion of alcohol during pregnancy. Caregivers may also fear that legal action will be taken against them if physical or drug abuse is discovered to be part of the patient's case history.

- Realize that parents or patients may not reveal significant diagnostic information because they may be unaware of what conditions are *significant*. Unless an anomaly produces a problem for the patient, he or she may never relate that anomaly to a genetic syndrome or systemic disease process. In such cases, the examiner must discover, point out, and question the occurrence of anomalous craniofacial features.

- Answer questions honestly. For example, if a parent asks, "Why are you asking me about the way Beryl's ears are shaped?" give them an honest answer. "You told me that Beryl has lots of ear infections. I noticed that Beryl has a receding chin and preauricular skin tags—little bumps that look like moles—in front of her ears. I am concerned that Beryl may have a hearing loss. I would like to give her a hearing test."

- Realize that some caregivers and patients will not accept your recommendations, even when those recommendations are sound and it would be in the person's best interest to follow them. This may be especially true if genetic counseling has been recommended. Refusal to seek genetic counseling often results when parents misunderstand the genetic counselor's function. A Miami University audiologist recently recommended that a patient with Waardenburg's syndrome have a complete hearing evaluation and receive genetic counseling. The patient refused the suggestion, saying that she "wanted more children, and she did not want a counselor telling her that she could not have more children." Although this patient was assured that the role of genetic counselor did not include directing parents whether or not to have children, she remained skeptical and refused to consider the recommendation.

Whether interviews occur before or after diagnostic testing, SLPs should be aware of factors that can confound the collection of accurate case history information. Shprintzen (1997) mentions denial and shame as elements that may cause caregivers to respond inappropriately to the examiner's questions. He contends that these emotions, while understandable in parents who have a child with a congenital anomaly, may cause the parents to delay, refuse, or misdirect care to their child.

Other, more practical issues may also impact diagnosis and treatment of patients with craniofacial anomalies. These include the patient's education and literacy level, regional or ethnic attitudes toward health care, and command of the English language.

Unlike families who request assessment from major craniofacial centers, the caregivers of patients identified through diagnostic screening may know little about craniofacial anomalies or their implications. Ignorance does not necessarily imply lack of intelligence or developmental delay. Family members may not view heterochromia iridis or prematurely gray hair as a cause for concern because they have not learned to associate these problems with serious conditions such as hearing loss. Family members may be aware of a child's unusual eye colors, but this may simply be accepted as "the way all the Smithfields' eyes look." Because families do not realize that a hearing loss and unusual eye anomalies are related, they may be concerned about the hearing loss but unconcerned about the eye anomaly. In such cases, interviews with family members have a two-fold purpose: data collection and patient education. Patient education can be difficult if family members are unable to read or if they speak English as a second language. Literacy issues are discussed in detail in Chapter Six.

Reviewing the patient's previous medical information before the diagnostic session can also provide focus and direction to the diagnostic process and prevent collection of redundant information. Although it is tempting to accept information in medical reports at face value, it is wise to keep all diagnostic options open. It is helpful to read the patient's medical records, separating facts from professional opinions. Knowledge about the patient's medical condition, about the patient's medication record, and about the history of previous diagnostic tests protects the patient's physical safety and allows the diagnostic session to proceed in an accurate and timely manner. Factual information, such as knowing that a patient is currently taking Dilantin, makes the examiner aware of medical conditions (in this case seizures) that may impact the diagnostic session. It also alerts the diagnostician to the possible presence of medication side effects, such as enlarged gingival tissue.

On the other hand, *opinions* contained in medical reports may or may not be accurate. Consider the following example from a dental report:

> Jimmy appeared to have problems understanding and following verbal instructions while having his teeth examined. His speech was difficult to understand. He was unable sit still for more than 10 minutes and was unwilling to allow his mother to leave the room. He appeared to be frightened by the noise of the dental drill and vacuum. *I believe Jimmy's behavior may result from attention deficit disorder (ADD) or cognitive impairment.*

The medical facts in this report include Jimmy's difficulty following verbal instructions, his physical restlessness, his unintelligible speech, and his fear of being left alone in an unfamiliar, noisy setting. The dentist's opinion that Jimmy had ADD or cognitive impairment is open to interpretation. As diagnosticians, it is useful for us to know that Jimmy may have trouble following verbal instructions, is restless, and fears being alone in an unfamiliar situation because these factors can be controlled during the diagnostic situation. Remember, however, that there are many reasons for the above behaviors besides ADD or cognitive impairment, including normal behavior of a very young child, sensorineural hearing loss, learned behavior from prior unpleasant exposure to a dental situation, and mild ataxic cerebral palsy. Treat medical *facts* as useful tools for planning diagnostic situations; treat *opinions* as suggestions that may or may not yield accurate information.

It is especially important to consider all diagnostic options while making visual observations. Remember to conduct *thorough* visual observations of every patient, even when current oral-facial examination reports are available. Methods of oral-facial examination vary from examiner to examiner, and even the most skilled observers may overlook important visual diagnostic clues.

Categorizing Diagnostic Observations

SLPs must be able to distinguish between anomalies that have implications for communication disorders and those that do not. It is, for example, easy for the novice examiner to mistake keloid scar tissue for preauricular skin tags, if those keloids are located in the auricular area. Preauricular skin tags may suggest the presence of conductive hearing loss; keloid scar tissue does not. Recommendation for audiological testing is warranted when preauricular skin tags are present; keloid scarring carries no implication for hearing loss or the need for audiological evaluation.

Differential diagnosis can be approached in at least two ways. Theoretically, diagnosticians could memorize all symptoms of every possible etiology and attempt to match each patient's diagnostic results to one or more of those etiologies. This diagnostic method would be a time-consuming process, even if it were possible to comprehensively memorize such material.

Obtaining an accurate diagnosis is more likely to occur when diagnosticians understand and categorize their observations. Understanding and comparing observations to categories of information is a feasible alternative to memorizing comprehensive lists of symptoms. Understanding an anomaly's observational significance makes it easier to narrow an initial diagnosis to one or two categories. Basically, craniofacial anomalies and their associated communication problems can be caused by trauma, disease processes, medical treatment, birth anomalies, or a combination of these etiologies. Subcategories for each general etiology also exist. Birth anomalies, for example, can be subclassified as malformations or deformations; medical treatment can be subclassified as iatrogenic lesions, side effects of prescription drugs, or results of cosmetic surgery. Etiologies may encompass more than one category, as in the case of genetically transmitted disease processes. To begin differential diagnosis, use the following basic guidelines to categorize the etiology of craniofacial anomalies. Notice how characteristics of each basic etiology differ from one another, and notice how they are alike.

Does the Anomaly Result From Trauma?

Trauma is probably the easiest basic etiology to diagnose. Trauma refers to any physical injury and can result from the birth process, accidents, self-inflicted injuries, and physical abuse. Table 4–2 summarizes basic characteristics of traumatic anomalies.

Table 4–2. Characteristics of Traumatic Anomalies

Background Information

- Patients often remember the traumatic episode that produced the anomaly.
- The patient or patient's caregivers may give inaccurate information if the anomaly was caused by child or spouse abuse.

Onset of Anomaly

- Onset is usually sudden.
- Onset may occur at any time during individual's life.

Location of Anomaly

- Traumatic anomalies may be located anywhere on the body.
- Traumatic anomalies often occur in isolation.

Symptoms of Anomaly

- Traumatic anomalies may be temporary.
- Traumatic anomalies are often painful.
- If the initial trauma interferes with subsequent growth and development of associated structures (e.g., untreated burns that fuse digits with scar tissue), the anomaly may become more noticeable over time.
- Traumatic anomalies may reflect the appearance of the object causing the trauma (e.g., circular scars from cigarette burns, semicircular bruises from bite marks).

Birth Trauma

Traumatic anomalies may result from the birth process itself or from perinatal medical procedures performed to assist the birth process. Although a variety of craniofacial traumas are possible, two are of particular interest to SLPs because of their superficial similarity to syndrome-produced anomalies: facial palsy and skull deformation.

Cranial nerve VII, the facial nerve, exits bilaterally from the parotid glands. Because of the glands' vulnerable location near the ear, the facial nerve may be compressed during the normal birth process or during a forceps-assisted delivery. If compression occurs, the baby may experience facial muscle weakness, drooping of the mouth, feeding difficulty, and inability to close the eyes (Thomas & Harvey, 1984). Because this situation usually occurs unilaterally, only one side of the face is generally affected. The situation often resolves spontaneously, but if permanent damage occurs, the child may have impairment of structure and function of facial muscles on the affected side. Similar symptoms can be caused by neurological conditions including Bell's palsy, cerebral palsy, stroke, and Möbius syndrome. Although patients with these conditions experience similar symptoms, the type of onset, duration of condition, and long-term outlook for each is quite different. Comparing birth history information, age of patient at time of onset, speed of onset, associated neurological problems, and spontaneous resolution of symptoms makes differentiating between birth trauma, birth defects, and neurologic disease processes easier.

Skull deformation during the birth process is relatively common and sometimes self-correcting. Because unusual skull shapes are also associated with delayed or early closure of skull sutures, knowledge of birth trauma may be useful for differential diagnosis of a young child with an unusual skull shape.

Accidents

Although anomalies resulting from accidental trauma may appear similar to birth defects, it is seldom difficult to distinguish between the two. The patient or the patient's caregiver usually remembers and can explain the presence of accidental traumatic lesions. Burns, contact with caustic substances or frozen items, electrical shocks, lacerations, bruises, and broken bones are just a few possible causes of traumatic craniofacial injury.

In ideal circumstances, the human body responds to trauma by successful healing of the traumatized area. Although the injury may heal completely, accidental injuries may produce permanent anomalies that directly cause or contribute to the development of communication disorders. The following case describing an acquired cleft of the hard palate is such an example:

Mrs. Thompson was a 60-year-old woman who was living in rural Mississippi when I met her in a prostodontist's office in Memphis. She had recently had her upper teeth extracted and was being fitted for dentures. When I examined her hard palate, I noticed a small, circular opening in the midline of the palate several centimeters anterior to the posterior nasal spine. The opening was surrounded by an area of scar tissue. I assumed that Mrs. Thompson wore some type of prosthetic device to obturate the opening in her hard palate, but this was not the case. She explained that the opening in her palate resulted from an injury she sustained when she was a 5-year-old child riding on top of a cotton wagon. While she was eating a piece of candy on a wooden stick, she lost her balance, fell off the wagon, and the stick holding the candy pierced her hard palate. Because medical help was unavailable, her injury was treated at home. Although her palate healed, the opening created by the stick remained, and her speech was noticeably hypernasal thereafter. When Mrs. Thompson entered public school, she was subjected to teasing because of her resonance disorder, and she experimented with ways to improve the sound of her speech. She discovered that if she positioned a blob of chewing gum in the palatal opening, she could speak without audible air escape. She continued to use this method to control resonance for the next 55 years, discontinuing it only when the prosthodontist designed upper dentures with a built-in obturator.

Self-inflicted Trauma

Craniofacial trauma resulting from accidents is often readily visible and easily identified, as in the preceding case. Self-inflicted traumas, however, may be so subtle as to be unrecognized by patients and medical professionals alike. Although SLPs employed in residential facilities sometimes observe obvious anomalies resulting from self-inflicted trauma in severely or profoundly mentally retarded individuals, such injuries are relatively uncommon. Nevertheless, diagnosticians who work with developmentally delayed or autistic individuals are likely to observe bite wounds to the lips, tongue, and digits of patients in their care at some time in their career.

In contrast, subtle self-induced traumatic behaviors may not be recognized as harmful by the individual practicing them. Self-inflicted trauma may result from dietary preferences or oral habits. For example, patients who enjoy consuming large quantities of highly acidic foods such as citrus fruits may develop loss of dental enamel over time. Localized abraded areas of dental enamel also appear on the teeth of patients who habitually chew toothpicks or bobby pins, or who brush their teeth vigorously with a firm-bristled toothbrush.

Dental enamel erosion resulting from rubbing cocaine into the gums or sniffing it into the nose is similar in appearance to dental erosion caused by eating highly acidic foods. The mixture of cocaine hydrochloride and saliva produces a strongly acidic secretion that is able to dissolve calcium from dental enamel (Krutchkoff et al., 1990).

Patients may also exhibit traumatic tooth enamel erosion resulting from contact with gastric contents from the alimentary tract. Tooth enamel erosion has been documented in patients with chronic bulimia (Rytomaa, Kanerva, & Heinonen, 1998) and in persons who have experienced alimentary disease, medication side-effects, drug abuse, and psychosomatic disorders over a period of years (Scheutzel, 1996).

Cosmetic practices may also produce trauma, such as keloid scarring resulting from the piercing of ears, eyebrows, and lips. Permanent bare areas on the scalp may occur in individuals who wear tightly braided hair over a long period of time.

In contrast to self-inflicted trauma, craniofacial anomalies resulting from birth defects often occur along lines of embryological fusion or organization—epithelial pearls on the midline of the palate, for example—or missing, ectopic, or malpositioned teeth adjacent to alveolar clefts (LeBlac & Cisneros, 1995).

Trauma Resulting From Physical Abuse

Trauma resulting from child or spouse abuse may be present, but unacknowledged by the caregiver (in the case of child abuse), or by the patient (in the case of spouse abuse). Although injuries from deliberately inflicted trauma may have little bearing on diagnosis of craniofacial anomalies, they have ethical and legal implications for the speech-language pathologist who encounters them. Consider the following case, in which child abuse ultimately led to legal action involving not only family members, but the health care provider as well.

Tiffany was a 4-year-old child who was receiving therapy for delayed language at a rural speech clinic. Tiffany's father had been previously arrested for suspected child abuse. At that time, Tiffany

(continued)

had been admitted to the local hospital with severe bruises to her torso and buttocks. Tiffany's father claimed that the injuries resulted from her falling from a swing. Because no direct evidence of child abuse could be produced, and because Tiffany herself was unable to describe what had happened, charges against her father were dismissed. One morning, during a routine therapy session, Tiffany's SLP accompanied Tiffany to the bathroom, helped her pull her shorts down, and helped her sit on the commode. In the late afternoon of the same day, Tiffany was again admitted to the local hospital, this time with life threatening injuries to internal organs. As before, Tiffany's visible bruises were located on her torso and buttocks. This time, a neighbor reported hearing sounds of a domestic struggle coming from Tiffany's house in the late afternoon. Tiffany's father was again arrested. During the subsequent trial, Tiffany's SLP was required to testify regarding the lack of traumatic injury to Tiffany's torso on the morning of the day in which the beating allegedly took place.

This incident is a reminder that as professionals SLPs must be continually observant of the entire physical appearance of our patients. Although this incident required the therapist to testify about a patient's normal appearance, it could just as easily have been a requirement to testify about the presence of traumatic lesions. SLPs should document visible evidence of serious physical trauma even if that trauma appears to have no direct bearing on the patient's communicative abilities.

Signs of physical abuse often have a characteristic appearance that differs from that of accidental injury. Multiple, circular-shaped burns may result from deliberately placed cigarettes; metal belt buckles may leave puncture wounds, as well as characteristically shaped bruises; and bite wounds may leave a unique, semicircular bruise, sometimes accompanied by punctures, lacerations, and localized swelling and infection.

Birth anomalies may sometimes be mistaken for trauma resulting from child abuse. Because of their location and appearance, Mongolian blue spots are sometimes mistaken for traumatic lesions. Mongolian blue spots (Figure 4–1) are areas of bluish skin pigmentation that look like bruises. These are often visible at birth on the trunk and buttocks of non-Caucasian infants and in Caucasian infants with dark hair. Mongolian blue spots are usually located in the same places where bruises from child abuse often occur. Bruises, however, appear suddenly on previously healthy tissue, are painful, and usually heal and disap-

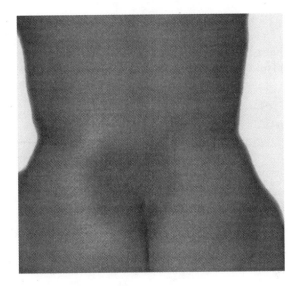

Figure 4–1. Mongolian blue spots on the torso of a normal African American infant.

pear within days or weeks. Mongolian blue spots are present at birth, are not painful, are not generally indicative of genetic syndromes, and usually fade and disappear within the first two or three years of life.

Tips for Diagnosing Trauma

- Ask the patient or the patient's caregiver about the origin of anomalies, even if the anomalies appear to be genetic. Scars resulting from surgical repair of accidental injury, for example, can look similar to scars resulting from repair of a cleft lip; however, the etiologies have quite different diagnostic implications. In a nonjudgmental manner, ask a question such as, "This is an interesting scar on Jimmy's upper lip. How did this happen?"

- Remember that patients with genetic syndromes can also have unrelated traumatic anomalies. Do not assume that all the patient's anomalies have a single cause. Areas of depigmented

(continued)

skin, for example, can result from burns, chemicals, deliberate application of cosmetic substances designed to lighten the skin, and lack of exposure to sunlight. These areas may appear identical to depigmented areas caused by syndromes.

- Observe the appearance of the patient's family members or ask to see family photographs. Anomalies resulting from trauma, deformation, or disease processes are confined to the patient; anomalies resulting from syndromes often occur in the patient's relatives as well.

- Read the patient's medical history carefully. Look for specific information about surgeries, hospitalizations, and reports of physical abuse.

In summary, differential diagnosis of traumatic lesions is not an SLP's primary responsibility. Recognizing traumatically induced anomalies, however, can hasten the diagnostic process by narrowing the list of diagnostic possibilities, ruling out genetic etiologies that might have implications for the patient's family members, and allowing diagnosticians to select an appropriate plan of treatment for communication disorders resulting from such trauma.

Does the Anomaly Result From a Disease?

Although SLPs are not responsible for diagnosing specific diseases, they do have an ethical responsibility to see that patients exhibiting symptoms of disease are referred for appropriate medical care. Table 4–3 summarizes general characteristics of disease-related anomalies. Because some diseases can affect the appearance of the craniofacial complex, it is important to distinguish between disease-related anomalies that have implications for communication disorders and those that do not.

Disease-related craniofacial anomalies that may have associated communication disorders include conditions such as Hutchinson's incisors and mulberry molars (congenital syphilis); cyanotic coloration of lips, fingernails, and skin (heart disease); and extensive tooth enamel erosion (chronic bulimia). Other serious diseases affecting the appearance of the oral cavity as well as the craniofacial region include herpes, HIV, sickle cell disease, lupus, and oral cancers. SLPs should be alert for the manifestations of life-threatening illnesses and should be prepared to make appropriate medical referrals, especially if the patient is not currently receiving treatment for those illnesses.

Table 4–3. Characteristics of Disease-Related Anomalies

Background Information

- If the disease has been diagnosed, the patient or patient's caregivers will be aware of the disease and its effects.
- If the disease is genetically based (e.g., Tay-Sachs disease, sickle cell anemia, cystic fibrosis) other family members may be affected.
- If the disease is progressive, its future effects can be predicted.

Onset of Disease

- Disease-produced anomalies may appear suddenly, as in the rash produced by rubella (measles) and the skin ulcerations produced by varicella (chicken pox).
- Diseases may occur throughout an individual's lifetime but may produce different effects depending on age of onset. Chicken pox in children, for example, produces wide-spread crusted vesicles that may scar. The same virus in adults or previously infected children causes shingles, a serious condition producing cranial or spinal nerve neuralgia as well as a characteristic pattern of crusted vesicles.
- Diseases acquired in utero may produce serious, teratogenous birth defects. Congenital rubella, for example, produces multiple defects of the central nervous system, eyes, and ears.

Location of Disease-Produced Anomalies

- Location depends on disease characteristics. For example, herpes zoster (chicken pox virus) causes skin lesions anywhere on the body; herpes simplex (cold sore virus) produces blisters and ulcers in the perioral area.
- The oral and nasal cavities are frequent sites of disease-produced anomalies.

Symptoms of Disease Processes

- Disease-produced anomalies may disappear when the disease is cured or has run its course.
- Fever and gastrointestinal symptoms frequently accompany disease processes.
- If the disease is progressive, its symptoms and the anomalies caused by those symptoms may become more noticeable over time.

Chronic allergies and otitis media are two disease processes that significantly affect the health and appearance of the craniofacial complex and can interfere with a patient's normal acquisition of speech and language.

Chronic allergies have short- and long-term effects on airway function, sleep patterns, linear growth, facial appearance, and the health of the middle ear, larynx, and upper airway. Communication disorders resulting from allergies include fluctuating hearing loss, voice problems, and hyponasality resulting from nasal airway obstruction. Chronically allergic patients often engage in frequent, habitual, and forceful nose rubbing. Such behavior is actually a type of trauma that if continued over time, may significantly displace the cartilagenous nasal septum, producing an asymmetric facial appearance and increased airway resistance. In addition, when nasal passageways are consistently occluded by swollen nasal membranes or deviated nasal septum, habitual mouth breathing will occur.

A chronic open-mouth posture, maintained over time, can prevent normal dental occlusion from occurring between the maxillary and mandibular arches. Normal dental occlusion must occur to prevent excessive vertical growth of maxillary dentition and the appearance of increased facial height (vertical maxillary excess). Vertical maxillary excess often occurs in combination with disorders of dental occlusion, such as open bite, tongue thrusting, and temporomandibular joint problems (Shprintzen, 1997). For these reasons, habitual mouth breathers should be referred to a dentist or otolaryngologist for differential diagnosis.

The high incidence of middle-ear disease in children with clefts has been recognized since publication of landmark articles by Stool and Randall (1967) and Paradise, Bluestone, and Felder (1969). Otitis media, irrespective of its association with craniofacial anomalies, can impair a child's acquisition of speech and language by causing repeated, fluctuating, conductive hearing loss. Children who have eustachian tube anomalies, as well as children with chronic allergies, are also at risk for otitis media. SLPs must always be prepared to refer such children to an otolaryngologist for medical treatment and to an audiologist for a hearing evaluation.

In summary, disease processes can produce temporary or permanent changes in the structure and function of the craniofacial complex. The ethical responsibility of recognizing disease and referring patients for appropriate medical treatment is compounded when the disease process has a direct influence on the development of communication disorders, as well as on the patient's quality of life.

Tips for Recognizing Disease Produced Anomalies

- Ask the patient about unusual appearance of craniofacial structures. If the patient is a child, or an adult who is unable to answer questions, ask the patient's caregiver for information. In a nonjudgemental manner ask, "Has Susan ever been treated for tonsillitis?" Or, "I notice that Jack has cotton stuffed in his left ear. Does Jack often have ear infections?"

- If the patient's caregiver is unavailable for questioning, ask to see the patient's current medication history. In educational settings, medication may be dispensed by the classroom teacher or the school nurse, depending on school policy. Look up the medication in a current *Physician's Desk Reference* (PDR), (Arky, 1998) to learn for what the medication is prescribed, as well as its possible side effects.

- Read the child's medical history. If current records are unavailable, follow your employer's policy for contacting parents or caregivers and for requesting information from the child's physician.

- Remember to request a copy of the child's dental records. Dental histories contain information about oral surgery, congenital dental anomalies, problems of oral hygiene, systemic illnesses, orthodontic treatments, cosmetic surgeries, temporomandibular joint problems, and a wealth of other useful diagnostic information.

- If current medical records are unavailable, contact the child's previous classroom teachers, SLP, and the school nurse to determine if the child has a long-standing medical condition such as heart disease, diabetes, leukemia, or sickle cell anemia.

- Some institutions protect confidentiality of patients who have HIV and AIDS. Be aware that HIV infection can occur in anyone, and familiarize yourself with the oral and otological symptoms of these disorders. Publications such as *The Otolaryngologic Clinics of North America: Otolaryngologic Manifestations of the Acquired Immunodeficiency Syndrome* (Tami, 1992) offer comprehensive descriptions of the most common manifestations of HIV.

- Congenital syphilis may produce Hutchinson's triad: blindness, deafness, and deformed teeth (Zatouroff, 1996). Recommend an audiological assessment for any child who has Hutchinson's incisors (small, widely spaced incisors with rounded or converging sides). Hutchinson's incisors are sometimes called "screwdriver teeth" because of their similarity in appearance to the tip of a screwdriver.

Sometimes it is not a disease, but the treatment of the disease that produces craniofacial anomalies. Minor anomalies, as well as temporary or long-term communication disorders, can result from medication, radiation therapy, and surgical procedures.

Does the Anomaly Result From Medical Treatment?

No medication or medical procedure is risk free. Characteristics of iatrogenic (medically produced) anomalies range from minor, temporary ones (such as scars resulting from removal of surgical tape) to serious effects that can impair the quality of a patient's life or are life-threatening. Table 4–4 summarizes basic features of medically produced anomalies. Like trauma, iatrogenic anomalies can often be easily identified; in fact, some medically produced conditions *are* traumas. Although minor medically induced anomalies are frequent following surgical procedures, they often heal readily with little lasting effect on the craniofacial complex or the production of normal speech and language.

SLPs are likely to encounter anomalies resulting from side effects of medication or from radiation therapy. Because such anomalies often appear similar to genetic anomalies, and because these anomalies sometimes interfere with normal speech production, SLPs must be prepared to recognize iatrogenic anomalies.

Table 4–4. Characteristics of Medically Produced Anomalies

Background Information

- The patient or his or her caregivers know the patient's medical history and can usually identify anomalies resulting from medical procedures.
- If medical treatment is in progress, future effects can be predicted.

Onset of Medically Produced Anomalies

- Medically produced anomalies may appear following an allergic reaction to medication. The oral and perioral areas are frequent sites of allergy-induced anomalies.
- Medically produced anomalies occur frequently following long-term medical treatment and in premature infants who remain hospitalized for long periods of time
- Medically produced traumatic anomalies may occur at sites where electrodes or surgical tape were attached to skin or at locations where IV catheters were inserted.

Symptoms of Medically Produced Anomalies

- Anomalies caused by medication may disappear or persist following discontinuation of medication.
- Anomalies caused by medication may appear years after initial treatment, as in tooth discoloration of wisdom teeth resulting from ingestion of tetracycline drugs during adolescence.
- Early head and neck exposure to high doses of radiation may affect the patient's linear height and facial growth.
- The appearance of the oral cavity structures and the perioral area is often changed by the body's response to prescription medication.
- Chemotherapy may cause temporary alopecia.

Side Effects of Medication

The effects of medication on communication disorders is a vast subject, which has been comprehensively described by Vogel and Carter (1995). Because drugs can have unwanted effects on muscle function, cognitive performance, and general health issues, SLPs must always remain open to the possibility that a given patient's symptoms may result from medication. Current descriptions of medications and their known side effects can be found in the *Physician's Desk Reference* (PDR). Antibiotics and seizure medications are of particular interest to SLPs because both produce effects that can be mistaken for genetically produced anomalies.

Patients with craniofacial anomalies often have associated neurological problems and seizure disorders. Several medications prescribed for seizures (as well as for other conditions) may have side effects affecting the craniofacial area. These medications include phenytoin (Dilantin); carbamazepine (Tegretol); and clonazepam (Klonopin).

Phenytoin is an anticonvulsive drug that is often selected to control tonicoclonic seizures. Side effects that could be mistaken for disease processes or craniofacial anomalies include development of a measles-like rash within the first two weeks of taking the medication, enlargement of lymph glands, excessive growth of body hair, and overgrowth of gum tissues. Overgrowth of gum tissues is a common and prominent symptom in children taking phenytoin. Compare the similarity between enlarged gum tissue and enlargement of tongue and facial tissues in a patient with Sturge-Weber syndrome (Figure 4–2). In this patient, tissue enlargement resulting from medication can be distinguished from tissue enlargement resulting from abnormal subcutaneous vasculature by comparing the right and left sides of the patient's face and oral cavity. The hemangiomas resulting from Sturge-Weber syndrome are often distributed unilaterally, along the path of the Trigeminal nerve. Seizure disorders are frequent in such patients. Ingestion of phenytoin has enlarged the gum tissue bilaterally, but has not affected the appearance of the right side of the tongue or face. These structures have become enlarged unilaterally on the left side by the underlying hemangiomas, seen here as darker areas on the patient's tongue, lips, and face.

Excess gum tissue may also obscure the upper portion of the teeth, leading to false conclusions about the size and appearance of dentition. Always check the patient's history of medication when in doubt about the relative size of teeth and gums.

Carbamazepine, another anticonvulsive medication, is also prescribed to alleviate muscle spasticity in patients with cerebral palsy, multiple sclerosis, and epilepsy. Side effects that affect the craniofacial area include skin rash, changes in skin pigmentation, hair loss, irritation of the mouth and tongue, and swelling of lymph glands. Clonazepam is

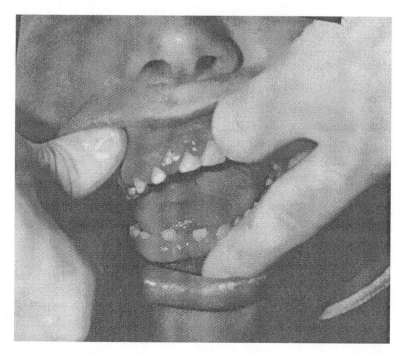

Figure 4–2. Intraoral view of a patient with Sturge-Weber syndrome. Note tissue enlargement on the tongue and gingiva on the right side of this photograph. Gingival enlargement results from ingestion of seizure medication. (Photograph courtesy of Edward Eiland, D.D.S.)

also used to treat seizures and may produce hypersalivation as a side effect.

Ironically, chemicals introduced into the drinking water to prevent dental caries can cause cosmetic changes in the appearance of tooth enamel similar to those of dental caries. Teeth are especially susceptible to exposure to high levels of fluoride in drinking water. As with ingestion of tetracycline, dental enamel may be discolored, and, in the case of fluoride, pitted.

Iatrogenic anomalies may result from almost any form of medical treatment. Most anomalies are temporary. Although large doses of radiation administered to the craniofacial complex of infants can affect subsequent craniofacial development, serious long-term negative effects on craniofacial structure and function are the exception rather than the rule. In such cases, the patient and the patient's caregivers are aware of the effects on craniofacial growth and appearance and can provide SLPs with relevant case history information.

Tips for Diagnosing Iatrogenic Anomalies

- Routinely review the patient's medical records before the diagnostic session whenever possible. Review the patient's current medication, and look up the side effects of those drugs.

- Ask the patient, or the patient's caregiver, about the origin of anomalies. Patients who have been taking medication for extended periods of time are likely to be aware of side effects.

- Remember that patients may be unaware of the effects of ingesting substances such as fluoride, iron, calcium, or other minerals found in local water supplies. These substances can substantially change the cosmetic appearance of dental enamel.

- Patients undergoing radiation or chemotherapy treatment may experience temporary loss of hair. Check medical records, or ask the patient or patient's caregiver about the patient's recent exposure to radiation.

In summary, SLPs should become familiar with the medical history of patients in their care and plan treatment for communication disorders with possible medical side effects in mind. Negative reactions to medications should be documented in the patient's records and reported to the patient, the patient's family, and the patient's physician. Because some medications can produce articulation or prosody problems in patients taking those drugs, the physician may need to adjust medication dosage to reduce or eliminate such effects.

Does the Anomaly Result from Cosmetic Practices?

The use of cosmetic techniques to enhance physical appearance has become commonplace. Treatments or devices are available to alter hair, nail, eye, and skin colors and to conceal blemishes and freckles. Surgical procedures can enhance the appearance of normal facial features and correct craniofacial anomalies. Orthodontic and prosthetic treatment can correct dental malocclusion and improve the appearance of unsightly dental enamel or malformed teeth. Other cosmetic procedures include application of tattoos and body piercing. Table 4–5 lists some characteristics of cosmetic changes.

Because such procedures are prevalent, it is wise to ask about cosmetic changes before beginning a diagnostic session. Although these

Table 4–5. Characteristics of Cosmetic Changes

Background Information

- The patient or patient's caregivers know and can identify changes resulting from cosmetic procedures.
- Patients may not know that cosmetic changes can alter the outcome of a diagnostic session. Patients may *not* volunteer information about contact lenses, hair dye, skin bleaching, or other changes from original appearance.
- If cosmetic treatment is in progress (e.g., application of dental crowns), future effects on the patient's appearance can be predicted.

Onset of Cosmetic Procedures

- Cosmetic procedures are initiated whenever the patient needs or desires them. Ethnic ideas of what constitutes attractiveness may influence use of cosmetic procedures.
- Cosmetic changes occur throughout life.
- Appearance of the oral cavity structures and the perioral area may be changed by cosmetic practices and by the application of surface cosmetics.

Location of Cosmetic Changes

- The following structures are frequently changed surgically: nose, lips, periocular area, facial skin, ears, and chin.
- The following structures are frequently altered with cosmetics, dyes, chemical permanents to curl hair, nail enamel, and tattoos: scalp and facial hair, facial skin, lips, nails, and eyelids.
- The following structures are frequently replaced by prosthetic devices: hair (replaced by wigs or falls); fingernails (replaced by artificial nails); eyelashes, teeth, eyes, and outer ears.

Appearance of Cosmetic Change

- Ideally, observers should be unable to detect changes produced by skillful facial plastic surgery, orthodontic work, or application of hair dyes.
- Contact lenses can often be seen if a light is shown directly into the wearer's eyes.

procedures are more likely to improve rather than harm the structure and function of the craniofacial complex, it is necessary to know what cosmetic changes have been made and why they were undertaken. Cosmetic changes that were made to conceal the effects of a genetic syndrome may mislead the diagnostician and result in an incomplete or inaccurate diagnosis. A patient with prematurely gray hair and heterochromia iridis may dye his or her hair and wear colored contact lenses to appear more attractive and "normal." SLPs who observe this patient without questioning his physical appearance may misdiagnose the patient as normal (or hearing impaired if a hearing loss is present) and miss the significance of the combination of prematurely gray hair and hearing loss. This misdiagnosis can have implications not only for the patient, but for the patient's relatives as well.

To provide an accurate diagnosis, SLPs must ask for a description or photograph of the patient's original appearance. In most cases, patients will not realize the importance of volunteering information about original hair or eye color or presurgical facial appearance.

Tips for Recognizing Cosmetic Changes

- Routinely ask all patients if they are wearing contact lenses. Ask if the contact lenses are a different color from original eye color; if so, ask the patient to remove the contacts during the oral-facial examination. The edges of contact lenses are usually visible when a light is directed into the patient's eye.

- Routinely ask all patients if they have had orthodontic work. Request copies of dental records.

- Ask patients about dental surgery and tooth extractions. Question the reasons for tooth removal (were the teeth ectopic, supernumerary, impacted?).

- Ask patients if cosmetic dental procedures such as crowns, bridges, and lamination of tooth enamel have been performed. Ask *why* such procedures took place.

- Observe the craniofacial complex for tattoos. The edges of the eyelids are a common place for application of permanent tattooed "eyeliner." Some ethnic groups tattoo the gingival margins. Ask about the patient's tattoo history.

In summary, patients whose appearance has been cosmetically changed may or may not have craniofacial anomalies. Suspect presence of birth anomalies only if case history or prior medical information so indicates, or if plastic surgery has been performed to alter the patient's original craniofacial appearance. If speech, hearing, or language problems are apparent, continue with routine diagnostic assessment. Recommend specific testing if evidence of velopharyngeal insufficiency or incompetence (VPI), hearing loss, voice disorders, or resonance problems are apparent. See information regarding birth anomalies below, and refer patients to a craniofacial center for specific diagnosis if conditions indicate.

Does the Anomaly Result from a Birth Anomaly?

The concept of a birth anomaly (formerly called a birth defect) can be misleading if the term is interpreted strictly to mean that the anomaly is present and visible at birth. Birth anomalies may actually occur throughout a patient's lifetime, and not all such anomalies can be visually detected. Some anomalies are internal, such as congenital malformations of the great vessels of the heart. Some anomalies are expressed as behavior disorders, mental illness, or cognitive impairment; and some, like sensorineural hearing loss, cannot be detected or measured through visual observation at all. Variability of genetic expression may further complicate the diagnostic process. As mentioned in Chapter 1, persons who have a genotype for a particular disorder do not necessarily exhibit the complete phenotype for that disorder. Finally, because many birth anomalies occur for the first time as new mutations, some patients may be the first persons in a family to have a genetic problem. In such cases, family history is of little use in diagnosing that person's genetic problem. Despite these diagnostic challenges, much can be done to correctly diagnose the presence of birth anomalies.

Keep All Diagnostic Options Open

It is tempting, but inaccurate, to classify every unusual craniofacial feature as a birth anomaly. To determine if birth anomalies really exist, observe the anomaly, and search for its *etiology* as well. Table 4–6 summarizes characteristics of birth anomalies. Compare these characteristics to those resulting from trauma, disease, iatrogenic anomalies, and cosmetic changes.

Learn to Recognize Normal Variations

The easiest way to begin to narrow etiologic possibilities is to ask ourselves, "Is this condition normal for this patient's age, gender, and race?" Novice clinicians are often startled by such normal conditions as a visible epiglottis in a very young child, epicanthal folds in young children of African descent, blue pigment along the gingiva of African American individuals, "strabismus" in Asian patients who have pronounced epicanthal folds, epithelial pearls in infants, and Mongolian blue spots on the buttocks of Asian babies. More often than not, these are normal features that warrant neither further testing nor diagnostic referral. In the absence of additional evidence, consider such "anomalies" normal features.

Some anomalies are minor birth anomalies that occur frequently, often in specific populations. These anomalies usually produce no negative effect on the patients' health. Such anomalies should be considered

Table 4–6. Characteristics of Birth Anomalies

Background Information

- Family members may recognize the existence, but not the significance, of birth anomalies.
- Family members may not recognize invisible birth anomalies (hearing loss, abnormal internal organs, behavioral problems) as genetic problems.
- Family members may be unwilling to acknowledge the existence of birth anomalies and may purposefully give the examiner misinformation regarding the anomalies in question.

Onset of Birth Anomalies

- Some birth anomalies (and some syndromes) can be detected before birth through amniocentesis.
- The odds of conceiving a child with a given birth anomaly are often predictable.
- Birth anomalies may or may not be visible and may or may not be present at birth.
- Phenotypic signs of a syndrome may continue to occur throughout life.

Location of Birth Anomalies

- Craniofacial anomalies often appear at sites of normal embryonic fusion (e.g., palatal shelves, skull sutures).
- Craniofacial anomalies often appear simultaneously in structures that develop from the same pharyngeal arch (e.g., outer ear and mandible).
- Craniofacial anomalies often appear simultaneously in structures that develop during the same embryological time frame (e.g., ear and eye).
- Craniofacial anomalies may appear simultaneously in structures that have an early embryological relationship (e.g., heart, left recurrent branch of Vagus nerve, and vocal folds).

Appearance of Birth Anomalies

- Some birth anomalies are considered attractive or sexually desirable (e.g., dimples in cheek, bright-blue eyes, gray central streak of hair in otherwise dark hair, minor cleft in chin).
- Some birth anomalies resolve spontaneously (e.g., Mongolian blue spots).
- Some birth anomalies become more noticeable as the individual matures.
- Birth anomalies associated with syndromes often have a characteristic phenotype.

insignificant, unless they occur in combination with other, more serious problems. Minor anomalies of little diagnostic significance include: preauricular pits in persons of African descent; nonelevated red capillary hemangiomas on the nape of the neck; clinodactyly of the fifth finger; supernumerary teeth; and syndactyly of the second and third toes.

Patients who have normal variations of facial appearance and patients who have isolated minor craniofacial anomalies in the absence of additional serious problems seldom need treatment for the anomalies, nor do they need to be referred for specialized medical diagnosis.

Place written documentation of minor anomalies in the patient's diagnostic report, and diagnose the patient's appearance as normal.

Rule Out Obvious Causes of Craniofacial Anomalies

Diagnosis of traumatically caused anomalies and of craniofacial anomalies resulting from medication have been previously discussed. If the anomaly is not a normal variation, is not cosmetic, and is not caused by illness, trauma, or medical treatment, the likelihood that the anomaly is genetic increases. Evidence to confirm a genetic etiology may be found in other family members, the patient, and the patient's case history.

Observe Family Members

Observing the family of a patient with anomalous craniofacial features can be a revealing process. Craniofacial anomalies caused by trauma and deformation are unlikely to be replicated in members of the patient's family. On the other hand, genetic anomalies, particularly syndrome-related genetic anomalies, are likely to be expressed to one degree or another in the patient's relatives. Unless the patient was adopted or has a new genetic mutation, it is useful to observe the appearance of as many of the patient's family members as possible. If you suspect that an individual has a genetic anomaly, try to arrange an interview with immediate family members. Use this opportunity to take a detailed case history and to observe the craniofacial features of the patient's relatives. Ask the family to bring photographs of siblings, grandparents, aunts, uncles, and cousins, as well as photographs of the patient at earlier ages. Clinicians can often make accurate, objective observations from photographs, particularly black-and-white photographs.

   If family members are unavailable for observation, it is still possible to obtain limited phenotypic information by asking the patient's caregiver to describe the appearance of siblings, parents, grandparents, or cousins. In a nonjudgmental way, say something such as: "Susie's eyes are an unusual color. Does anyone else in your family have eyes like hers?" Two different answers to this question may be especially revealing.

   If the caregiver says, "Oh, yes. Her father and her aunt have eyes that color. That's the Grayson family traits coming out in her," it indicates that the caregiver recognizes that the craniofacial feature is probably inherited, even if he or she does not understand the significance of the anomaly. This information also helps confirm the diagnostician's belief that a genetic problem may be present.

   On the other hand, if the caregiver says, "You know, our family has a joke about that. Susie doesn't look like anyone in our family. No one has eyes that color. My husband said if he didn't know better, he'd think Susie wasn't his child." This type of answer may indicate one of several things. It is possible that Susie's father *is not* her biological parent. Unless Susie's mother volunteers this information, we are unlikely to obtain accurate information about Susie's paternal genetic history. It is also possible that Susie's eye color is a normal genetic variation. Unless other phenotypic evidence is present to suggest a genetic syndrome, Susie is probably genetically normal. On the other hand, if additional anomalous craniofacial features are present, Susie's eye color may be a new genetic mutation, and she may be the first one in her family to exhibit craniofacial anomalies.

Observe the Pattern and Number of the Patient's Anomalies

Persons who have a syndrome, sequence, or association disorder often exhibit physical anomalies that occur in identifiable patterns. These patterns are not always externally visible, however, nor is differential diagnosis always possible based solely on the presence of such patterns. Nevertheless, several anomalies occurring in a specific combination are more suggestive of a birth anomaly than are isolated minor anomalies. Although opinions differ as to the number of minor anomalies that are suggestive of more serious problems, evidence suggests that the presence of three or more minor anomalies in one individual warrants evaluation for presence of a major anomaly (Jones, 1997).

In most diagnostic settings, the SLP's goal is to identify and document the presence of craniofacial anomalies and their associated communication problems, not to render a diagnosis of the specific syndrome, sequence, or association causing that problem. Syndrome identification is often difficult, even for members of craniofacial teams. Baraitser and Winter (1996), for example, report that most clinical dysmorphologists are able to diagnose only about 40% of the patients they see. Specific differential diagnosis of syndromes is best accomplished in a medical environment.

Consult Databases and Reference Books

Sometimes it *is* possible to identify syndromes by visual observation or to narrow the diagnostic possibilities based on visual observation alone. The craniofacial appearance of persons with Down's syndrome, for example, is generally recognizable because this syndrome occurs frequently and information about it is widely available from literature and media sources. The combination of anomalies associated with disorders such as Waardenburg's syndrome, Treacher Collins syndrome, and Robin's sequence are also unique and are seldom confused with other birth anomalies.

Although it is unrealistic to attempt to learn all diagnostically significant patterns of anomalies, it is a realistic goal to try to match diagnostic observations with descriptions of known syndromes. Comprehensive (and expensive) computer databases such as POSSUM and the London Dysmorphology Databases exist specifically for the purpose of assisting clinicians in making such matches. Although these databases are impressive, they are expensive and require specialized computer equipment and considerable computer literacy to operate them successfully. Web sites such as the one developed by the National Center for Biotechnology Information (www3.ncbi.nlm.nih.gov/omim/) also contain useful genetic information. This, and similar Web sites are discussed in detail in Chapter 7.

Persons who have limited access to computer sources can find photographs and descriptions of syndromes in atlases of birth anomalies. Some particularly useful atlases include *Clinical Syndromes* (Wiedermann & Kunze, 1997); *Color Atlas of Congenital Malformation Syndromes* (Baraitser & Winter, 1996), and *Smith's Recognizable Patterns of Human Malformation* (Jones, 1997). Although these atlases are expensive, they are available in medical libraries or through interlibrary loan programs.

In summary, suspect that birth anomalies may be present if a patient has no history of trauma, illness, or cosmetic practices that could produce such anomalies. Several minor anomalies occurring in the same individual are more diagnostically significant than is a single anomaly. Patients who exhibit a pattern of anomalies or who have family members who have a pattern of anomalies may have a syndrome. In such cases, referral to a craniofacial team may be necessary so that accurate diagnosis and team treatment of the patient and the patient's family can begin.

PATIENT DISPOSITION

Although referring patients for craniofacial-team evaluation is often a good treatment option, team treatment is just one of several choices available to patients with craniofacial anomalies. Other possible treatment options include no treatment; no treatment for communication disorders, but referral for genetic counseling; on-site treatment for communication disorders with referral to local clinics or hospitals for specialized medical care; referral to local or regional special-educational facilities (i.e., schools for the blind or schools for the deaf); or referral to local special medical facilities (i.e., endocrinology, burn, cardiac, or neurology clinics). SLPs should be familiar with local and regional treatment options and be able to assist in selecting the best treatment plan.

Health care providers (insurance companies) differ regarding reimbursement for specialized diagnostic testing. Many programs now require the patient's primary care physician to confirm the presence and etiology of birth anomalies and to make referrals for specialized treatment. In such cases, SLPs must work closely with the patient's primary care physician to make certain that the patient receives the specialized care he or she needs.

General Issues Regarding Patient Disposition

Following a diagnostic session, SLPs must review evaluation results and formulate a treatment plan if one is indicated. Patient disposition includes several basic steps, including preparing a written diagnostic report, explaining the diagnostic results to the patient and his or her family, making specific plans for treating the patient's communication disorders, and making specific referrals for specialized diagnosis and treatment.

Writing diagnostic reports is standard practice for SLPs. In addition to results of the intraoral evaluation, the report should contain a detailed, accurate, factual description of the patient's craniofacial appearance, with special attention to anomalous craniofacial features. Because information in clinical reports can serve as baseline data for future diagnostic assessments, it is important to include complete oralfacial descriptions, even if the patient's features are normal and no communication disorders are present. If the patient's craniofacial appearance changes, baseline reports can provide important information about the timing and nature of those changes. Maintain an objective viewpoint when writing reports, and use nonemotional language to describe observations. Sometimes photographic documentation is advisable, particularly if long-term treatment is planned and the patient's appearance is likely to be significantly changed as a result of this treatment.

SLPs should discuss diagnostic findings with the patient and his or her family before implementing treatment plans. Such discussions typically alert the patient to the presence of the anomaly, help the patient understand what the anomaly is and why it has occurred (if known), and suggest the anomaly's possible impact upon the patient and his or her family members. Communication disorders resulting from the anomaly should be explained, and recommendations for immediate and long-term treatment for them should be suggested. If results indicate that the patient would benefit from additional diagnosis and treatment by one or more specialists, then this issue must be raised also.

If team treatment is indicated, assure the patient or parents that multidisciplinary treatment is available, and give specific reasons why you think the patient would benefit from this type of treatment. Offer to arrange a diagnostic referral with a local or regional craniofacial team. Be prepared to provide family members with simple directions to the craniofacial center, suggestions regarding parking, and estimates of cost of service. Also provide specific names of contact persons at the cranio-facial center as well as e-mail addresses or telephone numbers.

If the family agrees to seek specialized treatment, the SLP should send a letter of referral, accompanied by a copy of the diagnostic report, to the appropriate professionals. This letter should contain specific rea-sons for the referral and specific requests for service.

Treatment Options for Patients With Traumatically Induced Anomalies

More often than not, patients who have traumatically induced anom-alies are aware of the anomalies and have received treatment for the ini-tial traumatic episode. Nonetheless, patients may continue to need information regarding the long-term effects of the original trauma, espe-cially if this trauma has produced noticeable facial disfigurement. SLPs should be prepared to take a proactive role in patient education, coun-seling, and acquisition of support services for patients with craniofacial anomalies. Guidelines for disposition of patients with traumatic anom-alies are outlined in Table 4–7.

SLPs, like members of the general public, sometimes hesitate to introduce sensitive issues for fear of embarrassing the patient. In well meaning efforts not to meddle in topics beyond their expertise, SLPs may err by not suggesting solutions for all the patient's problems. Although most SLPs do not have additional degrees in psychology, genetic counseling, plastic surgery, or other specialized disciplines, most know competent professionals to whom they may refer patients.

If the patient has craniofacial anomalies resulting from trauma, raise the issue of craniofacial appearance, and in a nonjudgmental way suggest treatment alternatives. Say something like, "I have tested Jill's hearing, language, and articulation, and they are normal. You mentioned that Jill has had large, lumpy looking earlobes ever since she had her ears pierced. Those lumps are called keloid scar tissue. Some people's skin reacts that way when it is injured. I understand that Jill has just turned 14. Teenagers often worry about their appearance. Has Jill ever said that she is bothered by the way her ear lobes look? Would you like to talk with a plastic surgeon about improving the appearance of her ears?"

Patients whose anomalies result from trauma may need assistance adjusting to the psychological aspects of living with, or living inside, a

Table 4–7. Guidelines for Disposition of Patients With Traumatic Anomalies

During initial diagnostic session:	• Place written description of appearance and location of anomaly in patient's diagnostic report. • Question patient regarding treatment of original traumatic episode. • Request copies of relevant medical records.
If patient has received or is receiving treatment for trauma and/or the anomalies resulting from it:	• Obtain and review medical records. • Obtain list of prescription medication. • Review side effects of prescribed medication.
If medical treatment coincides with treatment for communication disorders:	• Contact patient's physician and discuss implications of simultaneous treatment. • Consider impact of medical procedures on patient's communication skills, and schedule therapy accordingly.
If the anomaly's primary effect upon the patient is cosmetic:	• Suggest alternatives for cosmetic improvement. • Provide patient or caregivers with specific information regarding support groups for individuals with facial anomalies. • Remain sensitive to the patient's attitude toward his/her appearance. Suggest psychological evaluation or counseling if appropriate.
If anomaly's effects are cosmetic but extensive, and if those effects interfere with normal growth and development of the craniofacial complex (e.g., severe burns to face and neck):	• Recommend assessment and treatment by craniofacial team if patient is not already receiving treatment for long-term results of original trauma.
If anomaly affects structure and/or function of craniofacial complex:	• Conduct a diagnostic speech, language, voice, oral-facial, and audiological screening evaluation. • Follow up with specific voice, resonance, articulation, language, and hearing evaluations as indicated by screening results. • Schedule speech, language, or hearing therapy if test results so indicate.
Perform nasoendoscopic and/or videofluoroscopic evaluation if:	• Extensive intraoral anomalies are present (e.g., adhesions of faucial pillars, fistulae of hard or soft palate). • Neurological problems are present (e.g., velar and/or faucial pillar motion is reduced or absent). • VPI is indicated by presence of resonance disorders, facial grimacing, or presence of compensatory articulation errors.
If anomaly is primarily dental (e.g., abraded or discolored tooth enamel; missing teeth):	• Refer to dentist, orthodontist, and/or prosthodontist for cosmetic correction.

(continued)

Table 4–7. *(continued)*

If anomaly results from self-inflicted trauma:	• Place description of trauma in patient's report. • Caution patient regarding effects of continuing the behavior that is producing the trauma. • Make specific referrals to eating disorders clinic, drug rehabilitation units, or similar programs if warranted. • Follow up in six weeks to see if recommendations were implemented.
If patient is developmentally delayed and is engaging in self-inflicted traumatic behaviors:	• Explain results of self-inflicted trauma to caregivers. • Work with caregivers to develop a plan for stopping self-inflicted trauma. • Refer patient to behavior modification program.
If anomaly results from physical abuse:	• Follow your employer's guidelines for reporting physical abuse. • Place written description of traumatic anomalies in patient's files. • Consult your employer's legal advisor before photographically documenting evidence of physical abuse. • Recommend psychological assessment and/or counseling for patient and patient's family.
If patient requests help in stopping physical violence:	• Follow your employer's guidelines for dealing with physical abuse. • Most communities have battered women's shelters, safe houses, and other temporary living quarters for abused women and children. Become familiar with local community organizations that treat families who are subjected to physical violence; learn their referral policies, and make referrals accordingly.

less-than-perfect face. This is especially true for adult patients who have sustained facial disfigurement after a lifetime of looking "normal." SLPs should be prepared to refer these patients for psychological counseling if they appear to need psychological support. Local support groups or national organizations such as About Face can also play a crucial part in the patient's recovery from craniofacial trauma by providing group support from persons who have also experienced craniofacial disfigurement.

Generally, the more serious the original trauma, the more likely it is that a multidisciplinary approach will be needed to treat the resulting anomalies. Traumas occurring before craniofacial growth and development are complete may also require a team approach because injury to the developing craniofacial complex can interfere with subsequent normal growth and development. Long-term multidisciplinary planning may be necessary to treat the effects of burns, ingestion of toxic substances, facial lacerations, and broken bones.

Specialized evaluation is also needed if diagnostic results indicate that the patient's anomalies are affecting velopharyngeal closure or if the patient is exhibiting signs of velopharyngeal incompetence or velo-pharyngeal insufficiency (VPI). As previously mentioned, velopharyngeal closure can only be accurately assessed by instrumentational methods. If nasoendoscopic or videofluroscopic evaluation cannot be done on site and the patient is exhibiting signs of VPI, then the patient should be referred to a medical professional who has access to those techniques and is skilled in evaluating velopharyngeal closure.

In summary, SLPs should be prepared to document the presence of traumatic anomalies, institute appropriate treatment for communication disorders resulting from them, educate the patient regarding short- and long-term effects of trauma, and refer the patient for additional medical or psychological treatment if indicated.

Treatment Options for Patients with Anomalies Resulting from Disease

Diseases must be accurately diagnosed and treated, especially if they interfere with normal acquisition or production of speech, hearing, or language. SLPs must learn to recognize the presence of disease-related craniofacial conditions and refer patients for appropriate treatment. As with traumatic anomalies, education and counseling also form part of the SLP's responsibilities. SLPs must be aware of the special needs of patients with long-term or life-threatening illnesses, and must consider those needs when planning therapy.

Specific guidelines for disposition of patients with disease-related anomalies are presented in Table 4–8. The general responsibilities regarding disease-related craniofacial anomalies are essentially identical to those for anomalies caused by trauma. Disease processes differ from trauma, however, in that diseases sometimes recur, have long-lasting effects on the patient's general health, and, if left untreated, can sometimes lead to death or permanent disability.

Although SLPs are not responsible for diagnosing and treating diseases, it is their responsibility to refer patients to a physician. This is particularly true if, as with allergies and otitis media, the disease significantly affects the patient's communication skills.

Because parents may be unaware that "minor" conditions, such as allergies and otitis media, have serious effects on speech, language, and hearing, SLPs should be prepared to educate caregivers on these subjects. SLPs practicing in school environments are all too familiar with children who are sent to school (and to speech therapy) with discharging ears and otorea. Because otitis media is, from the parent's point of

Table 4–8. Guidelines for Disposition of Patients With Disease-Related Anomalies

If patient is being observed for the first time:	• Obtain and review medical records in advance of diagnostic session. Note presence of disease and medication prescribed for it.
If patient has anomalies secondary to a disease process (e.g., Hutchinson's triad/ congenital syphilis):	• Place written description of anomaly in patient's clinical diagnostic report. • Review medical records and question patient or caregivers about prior treatment. • Refer patient to physician for diagnosis and treatment of disease.
If anomaly's primary effect is cosmetic (e.g., discolored tooth enamel secondary to antibiotic therapy):	• Place written description of anomaly in patient's diagnostic report. • Inform patient or patient's caregiver of corrective measures to improve cosmetic appearance. • Make appropriate referrals if patient requests cosmetic treatment.
If anomaly affects function of craniofacial structures (e.g., allergies, hyponasal resonance and voice disorders):	• Make appropriate referrals to physician. • Advise patient that treatment of medical condition may improve or resolve communication disorder (if it will), or that failure to treat medical condition may interfere with progress in resolving communication disorder (if it will). • Schedule speech, voice, and language therapy if appropriate.
If patient has otitis media:	• Inform caregivers about effects of otitis media on general health, hearing, and language acquisition. • Refer patient to otolaryngologist for medical treatment. • Refer patient to audiologist for complete threshold evaluation if audiological screening results so indicate. • Follow up in six weeks to see if recommendations are followed.
If patient's tonsils look swollen, inflamed, or infected:	• Refer patient to otolaryngologist for diagnosis and treatment
If patient is a chronic mouthbreather:	• Refer patient to otolaryngologist. • Question patient or caregivers about history of allergies. • Make referral to allergist if indicated.
If patient has periodontal disease or dental caries:	• Inform patient or caregivers about the impact of dental hygiene on health. • Refer patient to dentist. • Follow up to see that recommendations have been carried out.
If patient has history of seizure disorders:	• Obtain complete medical records and list of current medications. • Discuss protocol for assisting patient in the event that a seizure occurs during therapy. • Be sure that the name of patient's neurologist, a list of patient's medication, and the patient's hospital preference are noted in patient's files.
If prescription medication appears to affect production of voice, resonance, or articulation, or if patient experiences tinnitus or change in hearing ability following administration of medication:	• Contact patient's physician immediately. • Document changes and circumstances under which they occurred. • Develop a working relationship with patient's physician when long-term prescription medication is administered, particularly for seizures, neurological disease processes, and diseases requiring treatment with ototoxic drugs.

view, not life threatening, they may consider it "just an earache," or "just Mary's allergies making her sick." Parent counseling is often necessary so the child can be effectively treated and the long-term effects of the disease minimized.

Counseling is a two-way street, of course, and the information exchanged often benefits the SLP as much as the parent. Always request a conference with parents when patients have a life-threatening illness, even if that illness does not directly affect the patient's communication skills. Be sure that a record of the patient's current medication and special needs is included in his or her file, along with names and telephone numbers of physicians and emergency care professionals.

Remain alert to the possible side effects of medical treatment. Persons taking ototoxic medications should have a baseline audiometric evaluation, preferably before the medication is administered and at appropriate intervals thereafter. Side effects of medication should be reported to the parent, the school nurse (if applicable), and the patient's physician when those effects are noted.

Just as patients who have craniofacial anomalies resulting from trauma may need direction and support in dealing with those anomalies, so may patients with long-term or life-threatening illnesses. Be aware of support services for specific diseases and inform patients of community support resources.

In summary, prepare to document the presence of disease-related craniofacial anomalies, refer the patient for appropriate diagnosis and treatment of disease processes, and monitor the effects of the disease process and the medication prescribed for it. If treatment for the disease involves medication or practices that impact the development of speech, hearing, or language skills, establish and maintain contact with the patient's primary care physician over the course of treatment. Remember that the patient and caregivers may be unaware of the disease's effects on the patient's communication skills. Prepare to provide appropriate counseling and information services and to refer the patient to support groups and additional information sources as needed.

Treatment Options for Patients With Anomalies Resulting From Cosmetic Practices

Generally, anomalies caused by cosmetic practices are of concern only in that they may be mistaken for birth anomalies, conceal true birth anomalies, or produce long-term harmful effects on the patient practicing those cosmetic techniques.

Table 4–9 provides guidelines for disposition of patients with cosmetically produced anomalies. Unlike anomalies produced by trauma or diseases, anomalies produced by cosmetic practices may go unnoticed. Because many people are accustomed to enduring a certain amount of discomfort in order to enhance their appearance, long-term side effects may be accepted as the cost of looking attractive. In any event, SLPs should remember to routinely question patients about use of cosmetic practices that could interfere with detection of craniofacial anomalies.

Referrals are sometimes necessary when patients request information about reversing the effects of a cosmetic practice, such as removing a tattoo. More rarely, a cosmetic practice may directly affect speech production, as in the effect of tongue piercing on articulation production. In such cases, appropriate counseling and treatment should be scheduled.

In short, cosmetic practices form a minor but important part of craniofacial diagnosis and treatment. Remain alert for cosmetic practices that may conceal birth anomalies, and prepare to counsel patients on the effects of cosmetic changes to the craniofacial area.

Treatment Options for Patients With Birth Anomalies

Although most SLPs do not have specialized training in genetics, genetic counseling, or syndrome identification, they are still responsible for

Table 4–9. Guidelines for Disposition of Patients With Cosmetically Produced Anomalies

If patient is being observed for the first time:	• Question patient about cosmetic practices that may affect accurate craniofacial observation (e.g., use of hair dye, contact lenses, artificial fingernails). • Place written description of cosmetic practice in diagnostic report.
If the cosmetic practice has long-term negative effects (e.g., tight hairbraiding/traction alopecia):	• Counsel patient about effects of continued use of cosmetic practice.
If patient expresses desire to reverse the effects of a cosmetic practice (e.g., remove tattoos, change appearance previously altered by plastic surgery):	• Make appropriate referrals to physician or plastic surgeon.
If patient's articulation, resonance, voice, or facial appearance could benefit from facial plastic surgery (e.g., plastic surgery to correct deviated nasal septum and improve nasal resonance):	• Inform patient of ways in which surgery could be beneficial (e.g., improved breathing, improved sleep patterns, and acquisition of normal resonance).

identifying the presence of birth anomalies and understanding the implications of those anomalies. They must also develop treatment plans for communication disorders resulting from those anomalies, discuss treatment options with the patient's family, and make appropriate referrals for specialized or team treatment. Specific guidelines for the disposition of patients with birth anomalies are presented in Table 4–10.

In theory, craniofacial teams represent the most effective way to diagnose and treat patients with craniofacial anomalies. As Middleton and Pannbacker (1997) observed, craniofacial teams are advantageous because they provide higher quality care at a lower cost, utilize a comprehensive approach to patient care, offer the convenience of interacting with a number of specialists during one appointment, and prevent duplication of services. Taken together, these advantages increase the likelihood of insurance reimbursement. That being the case, it might seem logical to immediately refer all patients who have birth anomalies to the closest craniofacial team and let the team members assume responsibility for the patient thereafter.

Before doing so, however, other factors must be considered. These factors include the quality and composition of the craniofacial team, the severity of the birth anomalies, and the family's preferences regarding medical treatment.

Quality and Composition of the Craniofacial Team

Although it is appropriate to think that team assessment is the most effective way to treat patients with craniofacial anomalies, there is currently no research to support this belief (Moller, 1993; Shprintzen, 1995). Because there is considerable variation in the number, quality, and professional expertise of craniofacial team members, SLPs should know as much about the craniofacial team as possible and be reasonably certain that the services needed can be provided by that team. The following example describes a child who was an ideal candidate for team treatment, but not by the craniofacial team nearest his home town.

Tom was born to a healthy mother following an uncomplicated pregnancy and delivery. His birth statistics were normal, and he experienced no perinatal health problems. He did, however, have a small jaw, a malformed left auricle, and a skin tag located between the left auricle and the left angle of his mouth. The physi-

(continued)

Table 4–10. Guidelines for Disposition of Patients With Birth Anomalies

If patient has been previously diagnosed or is receiving treatment:	• Obtain and review treatment records, preferably before initial diagnostic session begins.
During initial diagnostic session:	• Place written description of appearance and location of anomalies in patient's diagnostic report.
	• Question patient or patient's caregivers about origin of anomalies. Discuss family history of similar anomalies.
	• Contact individuals who are treating anomalies and discuss implications for simultaneous treatment of communication disorders.
	• Consider impact of medical procedures on patient's communication skills and schedule speech and/or language therapy accordingly.
If patient's physical appearance is substantially affected:	• Suggest alternatives for cosmetic improvement.
	• Provide patient or caregivers with specific information regarding support groups for individuals with facial anomalies.
If effects on growth, development structure or function of the craniofacial complex are expected (e.g., Möebius syndrome, Treacher Collins syndrome, Apert's syndrome):	• Recommend assessment and treatment by craniofacial team if patient is not already receiving team treatment.
	• Inform patient or patient's caregivers of specific support groups and services.
	• Perform comprehensive language, voice, resonance, oral-facial, and audiological evaluation.
	• Follow up with specific in-depth voice, resonance, articulation, language, and hearing therapy as indicated by initial results.
If patient has intraoral anomalies including neurological problems, fistulae, overt or submucous clefts:	• Recommend nasoendoscopic evaluation, videofluoroscopic evaluation, or both.
If VPI is suspected based on presence of such symptoms as resonance disorders, hoarse voice quality, facial grimacing, or use of compensatory articulation errors:	• Recommend nasoendoscopic evaluation, videofluoroscopic evaluation, or both.
If nasal regurgitation occurs while patient is eating or drinking:	• Recommend nasoendoscopic evaluation, videofluoroscopic evaluation, or both.
If patient has normal communication skills but a phenotype indicative of a syndrome:	• Question caregivers on family history of birth anomalies.
	• Refer family to a genetic counselor or a craniofacial team.
	• Refer patient to craniofacial team if anomalies are diagnostically significant in and of themselves (e.g., single central incisor/holoprosencephaly).

Table 4–10. *(continued)*

If patient has normal communication skills but anomalies that affect other body systems (e.g., internal organs, eyes, nervous system):	• Refer to appropriate professional for specific diagnosis of disorder (e.g., ophthalmologist, neurologist). • Refer patient to a craniofacial team if the appropriate specialists are members of the team, the patient appears to have a syndrome, or if anomalies affect craniofacial structure or function.
If the patient has minor birth anomalies and hearing loss:	• Refer to craniofacial team if an audiologist is a team member. • If craniofacial team does not have an audiologist, recommend thorough audiology diagnostic assessment, followed by referral to craniofacial team if hearing loss appears to have genetic component.
If patient appeared normal at birth but has recently lost some or all previously acquired skills (e.g., ability to walk, hear, communicate, speak, read, interact socially):	• Refer for specific diagnosis by specialist(s) in areas where skills have declined (e.g., neurologist, audiologist, psychologist). • Question family regarding history of similar disorders among family members. • Refer to genetic counselor if family history is positive for similar conditions or if genetic degenerative condition is suspected (e.g., muscular dystrophy).

cian at the small rural hospital where Tom was born reassured Tom's mother that the skin tag could be surgically removed and was no cause for concern. Tom passed an infant hearing screening examination, which was administered by a registered nurse, and he was sent home two days after birth. When Tom was 5 years old, he failed the speech and hearing screening at his local kindergarten and was retested by the SLP. Results of a threshold audiological examination indicated that Tom had a unilateral conductive hearing loss. An oral-facial exam revealed microtia of the left auricle and a small external auditory meatus. Tom's mandible appeared small, and his profile was retrognathic. Intraoral structures looked normal, but velar mobility was limited. Tom's articulation and language were age appropriate, although his conversational speech sounded hypernasal. After reviewing his medical records, the SLP noticed that Tom had undergone plastic surgery to remove the preauricular skin tag the previous year. When Tom's mother was questioned about the surgery, she assured the SLP that the family was not concerned about Tom's appearance, because "he looks just like his Uncle James." Further questioning revealed that Uncle James had a small jaw, a hearing loss, and absence of his lower eyelashes. Because Tom's phenotype and family history

(continued)

were suggestive of Treacher Collins syndrome, and because initial findings suggested the presence of VPI and hearing loss, the SLP believed that evaluation by a craniofacial team would be beneficial. The nearest craniofacial team was located in a city 100 miles away, but this team made quarterly visits to a large charity hospital in a city only ten miles away to provide treatment for patients with cleft palate. The team consisted of an SLP, a plastic surgeon, and an orthodontist. Although radiology and nasoendoscopic assessment were available, the hospital had no audiologists or genetic counselors on staff. The SLP believed that genetic counseling and audiological assessments were crucial for treatment of Tom's condition, and she contacted the national office of the American Cleft Palate-Craniofacial Association to inquire about craniofacial teams providing those services. She learned that such a team could be found in a major medical center in an adjoining state. This team met monthly and had ten permanent members, including an audiologist and a genetic counselor. After consultation with the family and with Tom's pediatrician, Tom was referred to this team, whose members ultimately diagnosed him with Treacher Collins syndrome.

Specific information about location and membership of craniofacial teams is published annually in the Membership Team Directory of the American Cleft Palate–Craniofacial Association (ACPA). In addition to a geographic listing of craniofacial teams and their members, the directory includes a catalog of parent and patient support groups and individual contacts and a list of publications available from the Cleft Palate Foundation. To qualify for listing in this directory, craniofacial teams must have a minimum membership of a dentist, a plastic surgeon, and a speech-language pathologist, at least one of whom is a member of the ACPA. Beyond these minimal requirements, there are presently no guidelines for what composes an effective craniofacial team. Shprintzen (1995) suggested that the original craniofacial-team model described above may no longer be adequate because advances in technology and medicine have made it possible to detect problems that could not have been detected when the original team treatment concept was developed. His description of an inclusive craniofacial team includes representatives from 26 specialties, including ophthalmology, pulmonology, genetics, social services, nursing, nutrition, and computer technology.

Craniofacial teams, as their name implies, are ideally designed to evaluate and treat craniofacial anomalies, particularly those involving clefting and those affecting the long-term development of the craniofacial complex. Examples of patients who could benefit from team services include, but are not limited to, individuals who have multiple anomalies and exhibit signs of VPI, multiple craniofacial anomalies of unknown origin, normal physical appearance and VPI of unknown origin, or a phenotype suggestive of a syndrome.

SLPs must prepare to provide specific documentation supporting the need for team treatment to the patient's primary care physician and to the patient's insurance company. Because of third-party reimbursement requirements, successful referral for team assessment depends in part on the SLPs report-writing skills, his or her professional reputation, and the quality of interaction with members of the local medical community.

Type and Severity of the Patient's Birth Anomalies

Not every patient with a birth anomaly needs treatment by a craniofacial team, although at times it can be difficult to determine which anomalies require team evaluation and which do not.

Severity of Anomalies

The severity of the birth anomaly can provide direction for selecting the best treatment options. Table 4–11 suggests treatment options for specific birth anomalies, based on severity and diagnostic significance of the anomaly. Use this information as a *guideline* for treatment direction and remember that any birth anomaly, no matter how diagnostically significant, can vary considerably in its effect on a given individual.

Number of Anomalies

Multiple anomalies in one individual are cause for concern, especially when those anomalies are suggestive of genetic syndromes. Conversely, some anomalies are diagnostically significant when they occur in isolation (Table 4–11) and are also suggestive of syndromes. Patients who have multiple anomalies or significant isolated anomalies may require not only accurate diagnosis and treatment, but family counseling as well. Families of such patients should receive accurate information about inheritance patterns and the probability of transmission of the genetic problem to future generations. In most cases, this type of educa-

Table 4–11. Birth Anomalies Categorized by Diagnostic Significance

The following anomalies are usually insignificant when they occur in isolation; some are normal racial variations. Unless additional signs of craniofacial anomalies are present, or unless the anomalies are cosmetically unattractive, no treatment is necessary.

	Presence Suggests	Treatment
Intraoral Anomalies		
Dark, pigmented areas along periodontal edge in persons of African descent	Normal racial variation Dark, pigmented areas located on the gingiva away from the periodontal edge may indicate Addison's disease. Such patients should be referred to otolaryngologist or dentist for diagnosis	None
Epithelial pearls in infants	Minor anomaly	None
Visible epiglottis in child less than five years of age	Normal feature	None
Supernumerary teeth	Often familial trait	None
Fissured tongue	Normal variation	None
Short lingual frenum	Minor anomaly	Usually none; short frenum rarely interferes with articulation
Ear Anomalies		
Preauricular pits in persons of African ancestry	Minor anomaly	Threshold hearing test recommended
Protruding ears	Normal variation	Refer to plastic surgeon for cosmetic treatment if patient wishes to improve appearance
Preauricular skin tags	Minor anomaly	Threshold hearing test recommended for all ear anomalies, minor or otherwise
Minor variation in shape or location of auricles	Minor anomaly	Threshold hearing test recommended
Eye Anomalies		
Epicanthal folds in newborns, especially babies of African or Asian ancestry	Normal variation Normal racial feature	None

Table 4–11. *(continued)*

Other Birth Anomalies

Simple capillary hemangioma on eyelids, bridge of nose, upper lip, forehead, or nape of neck of infant	Minor anomaly	Reassure parents that this condition usually resolves spontaneously; cosmetic treatment available if condition does not resolve spontaneously
Clinodactyly of distal phalanges of fifth fingers	Minor anomaly often familial	None
Postaxial polydactyly in persons of African descent	Minor anomaly often familial	None
Syndactyly of second and third toes	Minor anomaly often familial	None
Overlapping of little toe over the fourth toe	Minor anomaly often familial	None
Mongolian blue spots, especially in persons of Asian and African ancestry	Minor anomaly	Reassure family that condition usually resolves spontaneously

The following anomalies are often diagnostically significant for genetic conditions, especially when several are present in the same individual. Thorough diagnostic testing and referral for genetic counseling are recommended. If ear anomalies are present, audiological testing is indicated.

	Presence Suggests	Treatment
Intraoral Anomalies		
Bifid uvula Notched hard palate	Submucous cleft palate	Careful intraoral examination: voice, resonance, articulation **assessment; nasoendoscopic exam indicated of VPI is suspected**
Cleft palate	Craniofacial syndrome may be present	Craniofacial team evaluation and treatment highly recommended; genetic counseling suggested; audiological assessment and otological evaluation strongly recommended
Hutchinson's incisors	Congenital syphilis Hearing loss, neurological, and vision problems may be present	Referral to physician; audiological evaluation; referral to ophthalmologist
Ear Anomalies		
Low set, slanting ears retrognathic profile	Suggests conductive hearing loss and first arch anomalies	Complete audiological assessment recommended
Types I, II, III microtia	Suggests conductive hearing loss	Complete audiological assessment recommended; **referral to otologist**

(continued)

Table 4–11. *(continued)*

Eye Anomalies

Downslanting palpebral fissures	Craniosynostosis, unusual skull shape, Treacher Collins syndrome	Genetic counseling; craniofacial team assessment and treatment
Upslanting palpebral fissures	Primary microcephaly, cognitive problems, neurological problems	Craniofacial team assessment; genetic counseling
Hypertelorism	Craniofacial syndromes	Genetic counseling; craniofacial team assessment if other anomalies coexist with this one
Hypotelorism	Brain malformation, insufficient brain development; craniofacial syndromes including Trisomy 13, holoprosencephaly	Refer to craniofacial team; neurological assessment suggested
Heterochromia iridis	Waardenburg's syndrome, Fuchs syndrome, Horner syndrome, Gansslen syndrome, Parry-Romberg syndrome, Bloch-Sulzberger syndrome, Neurofibromatosis, Nevi of iris	Genetic counseling; audiological assessment; referral to ophthalmologist
Megalocornea	Aarskog syndrome, Scheie syndrome, Lowe syndrome, Rieger syndrome, among others	Refer to ophthalmologist; genetic counseling and team assessment may be required, depending on presence of other anomalies

The following anomalies are very diagnostically significant, even when they occur in isolation. Craniofacial team evaluation is recommended, as is genetic counseling. An audiological evaluation is needed if condition is associated with hearing loss.

	Presence Suggests	Treatment
Intraoral Anomalies		
Single central incisor or congenitally absent central incisor	Holoprosencephaly, central nervous system problems, brain malformation	Genetic counseling; craniofacial team evaluation; cognitive assessment
Ear Anomalies		
Congenitally absent auricle	First arch anomalies	Complete audiological evaluation
Unusual hairline or absence of hair in periauricular area	Middle ear malformations, conductive hearing loss	Genetic counseling; craniofacial team evaluation if condition is syndrome related

Table 4–11. *(continued)*

Eye Anomalies		
Epibulbar dermoids	Cri du chat syndrome, Goldenhar syndrome, other ocular conditions	Refer to ophthalmologist; craniofacial team assessment may be necessary if condition is syndrome related
Coloboma iridis	Optic nerve anomaly, CHARGE association, brain malformation, numerous syndromes	Refer to ophthalmologist; craniofacial team assessment may be needed if condition is syndrome related
Lip Anomalies		
Lower lip pits	Van der Woude's syndrome	Syndrome is associated with cleft lip and or cleft palate; craniofacial team assessment may be needed; genetic counseling highly recommended; condition is familial
Vertical median cleft lip	Cleft face syndrome	Craniofacial team assessment recommended
Other Birth Anomalies		
More than 6 café au lait spots	Neurofibromatosis	Refer to physician
Assessory nipples	Kidney anomalies	Refer to physician
Preaxial polydactyly	Orofaciodigital syndrome Type II Trisomy 18	Craniofacial team evaluation may be necessary

tion is best provided by a genetic counselor. Genetic counselors can be found in most major medical centers. Although genetic counselors are sometimes members of craniofacial teams, others are employed in specialized medical facilities that diagnose and treat genetic disorders.

Hearing Loss

Patients who have birth anomalies and hearing loss require immediate audiological assessment and treatment, irrespective of whether the hearing loss was produced by the birth anomalies. Because hearing loss is an invisible problem, it may remain undetected or untreated until its effects appear as delayed language, articulation disorders, or poor academic performance. Left untreated, hearing loss can negatively impact speech and language development and, in some cases, the health of the person experiencing the loss. Hereditary hearing loss, as previously mentioned, can affect not only the person experiencing the hearing loss, but other family members and future generations of family members.

For these reasons, it is absolutely essential that patients with suspected hearing loss or with genetic syndromes in which hearing loss is a feature receive early evaluation and treatment by an audiologist or an otologist. Patients who receive treatment from a craniofacial team that does not have audiological services should be referred for additional specialized evaluation and management of the hearing loss and the problems resulting from it.

Family's Preference for Patient Disposition

Treatment plans and referrals, no matter how accurate, are useless if the patient or the patient's family refuses to accept and follow them. The same factors that interfere with obtaining accurate case history information may also affect implementation of treatment plans. Emotions such as shame, denial, guilt, and fear can delay or prevent timely treatment. Religious beliefs and cultural ideas regarding medical treatment may affect the ultimate outcome of treatment plans as well. Conflicts about choice and timing of medical care may arise among family members. If family members differ significantly in their attitude toward the patient's condition, treatment may be delayed or withheld altogether, as in the following case of a child with vision and hearing problems.

Shortly after Beryl was delivered, the attending physician noticed that she had unusual facial features, including wide-set eyes, down-turned mouth, and a small jaw. The physician concluded that these features were not sufficiently unusual as to cause concern. By the time Beryl was 5 years old, however, it was obvious that she was visually impaired and had delayed language skills. Speech, hearing, and vision examinations were conducted at a local children's hospital, and Beryl was diagnosed with language delay, articulation problems, and a bilateral severe sensorineural hearing loss. In addition, eye examinations revealed that Beryl was legally blind. Because Beryl's hearing and vision loss had no readily apparent cause and because her facial features were unusual, a genetic evaluation was recommended. Beryl's parents disagreed about the need for genetic evaluation but, on her own initiative, Beryl's mother consulted a counselor at a local genetic clinic. Although a karyotype was made, blood samples taken, and a family pedigree constructed, results revealed no specific etiology for Beryl's birth anomalies. The genetic counselor was a consultant for the State School for the Blind, and she was aware of a special research project underway at this school. She informed Beryl's mother that if Beryl were enrolled as a subject in this study, she would be qualified to receive free hearing aids and eyeglasses and to receive rehabilitative training for her vision and language problems. Although Beryl's mother was eager to take advantage of this opportunity, Beryl's father refused to consider it because he "didn't want Beryl to go to school with a bunch of dummies." Beryl returned to her local kindergarten where she received speech and language therapy twice weekly and special training sessions for physically challenged children. Beryl's father remained adamant regarding hearing-aid fittings and became verbally abusive each time the subject of Beryl's hearing loss was raised. Beryl's mother consulted a marriage counselor and is presently contemplating divorce.

Although this case represents an extreme example of denial leading to delayed and ineffective treatment, opposition to treatment plans by one or more family members of patients with birth anomalies is not uncommon. In many cases, time, coupled with patient education, can facilitate treatment plans. See the following chapter for specific information on evaluating and preparing materials for patient education.

SUMMARY

Understanding the implications of visual observations assists in differential diagnosis and patient disposition. Comparing background information to visual observations and results of diagnostic testing allows SLPs to categorize their diagnostic findings and choose the most likely etiology for the patient's anomalies.

Anomalies may result from trauma, disease processes, medical procedures, cosmetic practices, or birth anomalies. SLPs can narrow their diagnostic choices by ruling out obvious causes of anomalies, observing members of the patient's family, observing the pattern and number of the patient's anomalies, and consulting reference materials.

Treatment for patients with craniofacial anomalies may include assessment by a craniofacial team or appropriate specialists including audiologists, plastic surgeons, and genetic counselors. While craniofacial team assessment is appropriate for patients with craniofacial anomalies, genetic syndromes, and anomalies producing long-term effects, the SLP must be careful to match the craniofacial team with the needs of a given patient. Variability in composition and skills of craniofacial team members may occasionally make team treatment inappropriate. In such cases, SLPs must be prepared to refer the patient to alternative sources for diagnosis and treatment. In any case, treatment options must be accepted and followed by the patient and the patient's caregivers if treatment is to be successful.

REFERENCES

Arky, R. (1998). *Physician's desk reference.* Montvale, NJ: Medical Economics Company, Inc.

Baraitser, M., & Winter, R. M. (1996). *Color atlas of congenital malformation syndromes.* London: Mosby-Wolfe.

Emerick, L., & Haynes, W. (1986). *Diagnosis and evaluation in speech pathology.* Englewood Cliffs, NJ: Prentice Hall.

Jones, K. L. (1997). *Smith's recognizable patterns of human malformation.* Philadelphia: W. B. Saunders Co.

Krutchkoff, D. J., Eisenberg, E., O'Brien, J. E., & Ponzillo, J. J. (1990). Cocaine induced dental erosions. *The New England Journal of Medicine, 322,* 1408.

LeBlanc, E., & Cisneros, G. (1995). The dynamics of speech and orthodontic management in cleft lip and palate. In R. J. Shprintzen & J. Bardach (Eds.), *Cleft palate speech management* (pp. 305–325). St. Louis, MO: Mosby.

Middleton, G. F., & Pannbacker, M. (1997). *Cleft palate and related disorders.* Bisbee, AZ: Imaginart.

Moller, K. T. (1993). Interdisciplinary team approach: Issues and procedures. In Moller, K. T. & Starr, C. D. (Eds.), *Cleft palate: Interdisciplinary issues and treatment* (pp. 1–20). Austin, TX: PRO-ED.

Morris, H. L., & Hall, P. K. (1994). The clinical history. In J. B. Tomblin, H. L. Morris & D. L. Spriestersbach (Eds.), *Diagnosis in speech-language pathology* (pp. 53–64). San Diego, CA: Singular Publishing Group.

Paradise, J. L., Bluestone, C. D., & Felder, H. (1969). The universality of otitis media in 50 infants with cleft palate. *Pediatrics, 44,* 35–42.

Peterson, H., & Marquardt, T. (1994). *Appraisal and diagnosis of speech and language disorders.* Englewood Cliffs, NJ: Prentice Hall.

Rytomaa, I., Jarvinen, V., Kanerva, R., & Heinonen, O. (1998). Bulimia and tooth erosion. *Acta Odontologica Scandinavica, 56,* 36–40.

Scheutzel, P. (1996). Etiology of dental erosion-intrinsic factors. *European Journal of Oral Sciences, 104,* 178–90.

Shipley, K. G., & McAfee, J. G. (1992). *Assessment in speech-language pathology: A resource manual.* San Diego, CA: Singular Publishing Group.

Shprintzen, R. J. (1995). A new perspective on clefting. In Shprintzen, R. J. & Bardach, J. (Eds.). *Cleft palate speech management* (pp. 1–15). St. Louis, MO: Mosby.

Shprintzen, R. J. (1997). *Genetics, syndromes, and communication disorders.* San Diego, CA: Singular Publishing Group.

Stool, S. E., & Randall, P. (1967). Unexpected ear disease in infants with cleft palate. *Cleft Palate Journal, 4,* 99–103.

Tami, T. A. (Ed.). (1992). *The otolaryngologic clinics of North America. Vol. 25: Otolaryngologic manifestations of the acquired immunodeficiency syndrome.* Philadelphia: W. B. Saunders Co.

Thomas, R., & Harvey, D. (1984). *Neonatology.* New York: Churchill Livingstone.

Vogel, D., & Carter, J. (1995). *The effects of drugs on communication disorders.* San Diego, CA: Singular Publishing Group.

Wiedemann, H. R., & Kunze, J. (1997). *Clinical syndromes.* London: Mosby-Wolfe.

Zatouroff, M. (1996). *Diagnosis in color. Physical signs in general medicine* (2nd ed.). London: Mosby-Wolfe.

CHAPTER 5

WRITING READABLE CLINICAL MATERIALS

Health care professionals create written materials for a variety of purposes, three of which are especially important to the observation of craniofacial anomalies. Written materials can be used to educate patients and colleagues, to document observations, and to create legal agreements between two or more parties. It is beyond the scope of this text to teach comprehensive methods of writing clinical reports, informational pamphlets, or legal forms. Those issues are addressed successfully elsewhere (see "Expanding Your Knowledge Base" at the end of this chapter). One issue however, deserves in-depth attention because it is seldom discussed, even in textbooks designed to teach clinical writing skills. That issue is adult literacy.

WHAT DOES ADULT LITERACY HAVE TO DO WITH ME? I DON'T TREAT ILLITERATE PATIENTS

Several years ago, a colleague and I attended a national conference on aging. During the conference, we conducted a random survey on the topic of adult reading skills. We asked approximately 30 conference attendees to complete a brief survey and were surprised when most refused to do so. When we asked why they were reluctant to fill out a one-page questionnaire, most persons responded by saying that the survey's topic did not apply to them. As one nursing home director indignantly stated, We don't have *that kind* of resident at *our* facility!

The director probably would have been shocked had he known the actual reading ability of the persons living in *his* facility. The results of a recent literacy survey of American adults are not only surprising, but alarming. In 1993, the National Center for Education Statistics conducted a study of adult literacy by randomly sampling a total of 26,000 Americans over the age of 16. Participants were required to complete a series of literacy tasks and were measured on prose, document, and quantitative literacy. Results were categorized into five levels. Each level encompassed a range of skills related to reading ability.

The lowest level, Level 1, described persons whose abilities ranged from being able to perform very simple reading tasks to being almost unable to perform any literacy tasks at all. During the survey, for example, some Level 1 readers were able to identify specific information in a newspaper article or to add a column of figures in a checkbook, while others had such limited skills that they were unable to complete the survey.

Level 2 participants demonstrated somewhat higher proficiency in that they could locate information in text, perform quantitative tasks that involved a single operation, and complete tasks such as finding a particular intersection on a street map. Level 2 readers often had difficulty performing tasks that required integration or synthesization of information from lengthy text.

Persons who functioned at Level 3 were able to read and integrate information from long or dense text or documents and to perform more difficult mathematical calculations. Examples of Level 3 tasks included using a bus schedule to determine the appropriate bus for a specific set of conditions, writing a brief letter explaining an error in a credit-card bill, and calculating miles per gallon using information on a mileage record chart.

Persons in Level 4 were required to demonstrate proficiencies associated with challenging tasks such as comparing metaphors used in a poem, using a table of information to determine the pattern of oil exports across years, and determining the correct change by using information in a menu.

Persons who functioned at the highest level, Level 5, were able to perform complex tasks. Examples of Level 5 tasks include summarizing two ways lawyers may challenge prospective jurors, using tabled information to complete a graph, and using a calculator to determine the total cost of carpet to cover a room.

Following analysis of survey results, approximately 90 million adults (47% of U.S. adults) were estimated to function in the two lowest categories of literacy skills. Of the 40 to 44 million adults at the lowest level, 62% had not completed high school, and 25% were immigrants. Fifty million adults were placed at Level 2 and had difficulty with higher reading and problem solving skills. Although older adults, minorities, and prison inmates were most likely to have literacy problems, young adults were also at risk. Young adults in the 1993 survey were less proficient in reading ability than those surveyed in 1985.

If the results of this survey are accurate, almost one in two American adults could be functionally illiterate. No matter what our employment setting, there surely will be at least a few of that kind of people in our daily environment. It is therefore necessary to understand the implications of functional illiteracy to provide accurate diagnosis and treatment to all our patients.

WHAT IS FUNCTIONAL ILLITERACY?

Functionally illiterate individuals are persons who have the minimal level of literacy development required to meet the normal demands of daily life (Heisel & Larson, 1984). Such persons can often print their name, read food labels, and calculate correct change at the grocery store. They are usually *unable* to make higher level deductions requiring comparison of written material or to perform simple mathematical calculations. Although they may be able to read a newspaper, they may be unable to summarize the contents of what they have read. Illiterate individuals will go to great lengths to insure that their condition goes undetected, even to the point of pretending to read therapy materials, diagnostic reports, and educational materials distributed by health care professionals.

Because the creation and distribution of written materials is a major part of diagnosis and therapy, those materials must be carefully prepared. If written material is to accomplish its purpose, clinicians must do two things: They must be aware of functionally illiterate patients in their care and be certain that written materials are readable for every patient.

Identifying Functionally Illiterate Individuals

Functionally illiterate individuals are, in the simplest definition, people who are unable to read. Categories of people most likely to be functionally illiterate include persons who:

- speak English as a second language
- did not receive a formal education
- discontinued their formal education
- did not or could not use their educational opportunities wisely
- received poor quality educational services
- are developmentally disabled
- have learning disabilities.

Because the above characteristics are often not readily apparent, it is not possible to identify literacy level based solely on an individual's age, physical appearance, or economic status. Illiterate individuals are present in every environment, no matter how prestigious the setting. Such persons teach in our school systems, serve in public office, care for our children, serve in our armed forces, star in major motion pictures, and win national sports events. Functionally illiterate persons are part of our clinical caseloads and are the family members of some of our patients. While we may not be able to identify all functionally illiterate persons in our care, we can be alert for behaviors common to nonreading individuals. Positive identification of functionally illiterate adults is difficult in part because illiteracy is an invisible problem and in part because illiterate persons prefer that the problem remains invisible. The inability to read has negative social consequences in our society because of the prevailing idea that illiterate persons also must be unintelligent. Few functionally illiterate persons are willing to reveal their reading problems directly because if those problems are discovered, embarrassment and loss of self-esteem can occur. The following case represents such a situation.

Some years ago, I sponsored a support group for individuals with laryngectomies. Mr. Brown, a financially successful farmer, had undergone a laryngectomy and later provided bedside counseling to recent laryngectomy patients. He was active in the support group and made inspirational speeches to community organizations. He also continued to perfect his esophageal speaking skills by reading words and sentences from practice sheets prepared by his speech pathologist. During the course of the year, the president of the local laryngectomy group retired. I encouraged Mr. Brown to campaign for this office. Mr. Brown was visibly reluctant and refused repeatedly, although he could see that I was puzzled and disappointed by his refusal. Finally, he explained his decision. His statement, I'm too stupid to do the paperwork was reluctantly modified to, I'm too stupid to *read* the paperwork. I was surprised and unbelieving. I didn't understand how someone who claimed to be unable to read could complete written assignments and read written material aloud during therapy. He explained that he took the written material home, memorized it with the assistance of his wife, and repeated it from memory during subsequent therapy sessions. I asked if he would like to learn to read and offered to enroll him in an adult literacy program, but he refused, saying he was too stupid and too old to learn.

Mr. Brown is typical of many nonreading individuals. Although he had a limited formal education, he had devised strategies for concealing his educational deficiencies. His family support system helped him function marginally in those areas of his life where reading was required. Far from being stupid, he was able to learn material that assisted him in overcoming the loss of his voice following laryngectomy and which helped him make a positive contribution to the community. His recovery might have proceeded more quickly and pleasantly had his therapist identified his reading problem and modified therapy materials accordingly. This is not as easy as it sounds.

Although Mr. Brown did not willingly admit to having a reading problem, he displayed subtle signs that could have indicated that literacy was an issue. Table 5–1 summarizes strategies that are indicative of functional illiteracy.

Not everyone who forgets to bring reading glasses to therapy is functionally illiterate, of course. A pattern of subtle behaviors is more indicative of reading difficulty than a few episodes of forgetfulness. Consider your clinical or educational setting for a moment. Are you working with someone who has never completed a written assignment in your presence, who always complains that the lights are too dim, or the print is too small to read? Does this person have a legible signature, or does he or she "write" in an unintelligible squiggle? If your facility requires patients to sign in upon arrival, does your patient often "forget"

Table 5–1. Coping Strategies Used by Functionally Illiterate Adults

To conceal reading problems, functionally illiterate adults often:

- "Forget" to bring their reading glasses to therapy
- Ask to complete written work at home
- "Don't have time" to complete written assignments
- Request that spouses complete paperwork
- Ask health care professionals to help fill out forms
- Complain of "tired eyes," "headaches," or "arthritis in my hand"
- Write illegibly or print in block letters
- Pretend to read magazines while sitting in the waiting room
- Deny problems with reading if confronted directly

to do this? If you answered "yes" to most of these questions, then literacy could be the factor governing your patient's behavior.

It is desirable, but not absolutely essential, to identify nonreading adults in our care. Even if such patients cannot be positively identified, just understanding that they are likely to be a part of the SLPs' caseload is sufficient reason for examining our written materials for readability. In order to do this, we must first understand what readability is, and how it is measured.

EVALUATING READABILITY OF WRITTEN MATERIALS

What Is Readability?

Many factors make written material readable. Some of these, including appearance, organization, and readability level of the document, are directly under the clinician's control. Others, like a patient's IQ, interest in a particular subject, or level of education depend entirely on the patient. Readability levels are usually computed by using one or more readability formulas. The results are expressed in terms of grade level or ease of reading.

Measuring Readability

Readability formulas have been used for decades to assess the degree of reading difficulty, and there are more than 50 formulas to choose from. Most formulas use average sentence length, the number of syllables per word, and the difficulty of vocabulary to determine level of reading ease. Grade level is often determined by counting the number of sentences and multisyllabic words in several random passages and by comparing these numbers to readability charts or tables. Hand calculation of readability level is a simple although tedious and time consuming process. It is faster and easier to calculate readability using the grammar check function in Microsoft Word Version 6.01 or higher for Macintosh or PC. This program provides information such as word count and average number of sentences per paragraph. It also displays the number of sentences that are written in passive voice, and computes readability of the document using four different readability formulas.

Using Readability Formulas Responsibly

An easy readability grade level alone cannot guarantee that a document is useful or educational. Moreover, motivated patients with minimal reading skills often successfully read material written at higher grade levels. Because multiple factors determine overall readability, readability formulas are most useful when used as an initial means of evaluating the readability level of existing documents. Clinicians must have reasonable expectations about readability formulas and be aware of their limitations. Table 5–2 presents guidelines for responsible use of readability formulas.

Readability levels provide a starting point for revising clinical materials. Although knowing a document's grade level is useful, there are other factors to consider when revising documents.

MAKING EDUCATIONAL
MATERIALS READABLE

Ideally, before writing or rewriting educational material, it is best to determine the reading level of the target readers. This process requires time, patient cooperation, and individual modification of teaching materials. Time and financial constraints make the process of determining every patient's reading level impossible in most clinical settings. For clinicians who do have the time, Doak, Doak, and Root (1985) have pro-

Table 5–2. Guidelines for Responsible Use of Readability Formulas

Use readability formulas for:

• Measuring countable features (words per sentence or syllables per word)

• Providing a starting point for revising existing written material

• Providing objective measures of readability level

Choose other methods to evaluate:

• Appropriateness of subject matter

• Accuracy of content

• Readability of graphs or illustrations

• Usefulness of information to the reader

• Legal documents

• Forms and charts

vided excellent guidelines for testing patients' comprehension of written materials.

For most clinicians, however, it is more feasible to determine the readability of existing educational material and to rewrite it at a preselected reading level, fourth-grade level, for example. Writing educational materials for functionally illiterate adults requires examining material from a new perspective, particularly when organizing information, selecting appropriate vocabulary, or creating illustrations and study aids.

Adults with limited reading experience may have difficulty understanding a document's content, even if the content is written at a lower grade level. There are several reasons for this. The most basic is that unskilled readers seldom associate written words with an underlying message. When asked to define what reading a book means, functionally illiterate persons often reply that "reading" means saying the words aloud without mispronouncing them. Initially, most unskilled readers make little connection between words on a page and the message that those words convey. When a message is perceived, it is likely to be a literal rather than an abstract one. Because functionally illiterate persons are likely to have difficulty making abstractions, they learn best from materials that have direct application to personal experiences. Table 5–3 summarizes factors that make reading difficult for unskilled readers.

Table 5-3. Factors That Make Reading Difficult

Unskilled readers may not be able to:

- "Read" the messages delivered by type style (such as italics or bold face type)
- Interpret slang, abbreviations, or idioms
- Extract relevant information from charts or illustrations
- Organize information into units
- Use study aids, such as glossaries
- Understand acronyms

Unskilled readers may ignore:

- Long passages of information
- Small print or elaborate fonts
- Multicolored text
- Foreign words or expressions
- Words written in capital letters
- Words written in cursive writing

Modifying Brochures and Pamphlets

Professional associations, hospitals, and clinics often allot substantial educational budgets for preparation of brochures and instruction sheets. In theory, these materials supplement the caregiver's instructions and allow patients to better understand their plan of care. In fact, educational materials are not always readable by the persons they are designed to serve. During a readability analysis of 18 pamphlets published for families and patients with cleft palate, Kahn and Pannbacker (in press) found the readability of such documents to range from elementary to college level, with the majority being written at high school level. Results suggested that although the pamphlets contained useful information, functionally illiterate persons might have difficulty accessing that information. In addition, the target audience and readability level of several publications seemed mismatched. For example, *Cleft Lip and Cleft Palate: Information for the Teenager Born with Cleft Lip, and/or Cleft Palate* (Cleft Palate Foundation, 1980) required a college-level education to understand the material. Other readability studies have found similar results for material about heart disease (Laidlaw & Harden, 1987), elementary-school health care (Frager & Kahn, 1988), and audiology (Kelly & Kahn, 1991, Kelly, 1996).

Keeping in mind that functionally illiterate persons are currently estimated to comprise 47% of the population of the United States, clinicians must ensure that materials supplied to patients are readable. Does that mean that all materials must be rewritten at the fourth-grade reading level? Not necessarily. Several choices are available for selecting educational materials for functionally illiterate patients. One option is to read the material aloud to the patient and then discuss the contents. This method is time consuming but allows us to form some idea of the patient's level of understanding and to answer the patient's questions.

If the patient's reading level is known, educational materials written at approximately that reading level can be selected for that patient. Too often, however, there are no easy adult materials available on specialized topics such as craniofacial anomalies. In such cases, we must either write our own materials or modify existing ones to make them easier to read. Regardless of which option is selected, clinicians can expedite the process of educating functionally illiterate patients by preparing readable materials in advance. Existing materials can be scanned into a computer and analyzed for readability using previously described computer-generated readability formulas. Materials with high readability levels can then be simplified using the guidelines in Table 5–4. These guidelines also apply when generating new materials specifically designed for functionally illiterate readers. Although it is usually more efficient to simplify existing documents than to generate new material for educational purposes, copyright laws must be respected. Because copyrighted material may not be reproduced or redesigned without permission of the author or authors, it is sometimes necessary to create new materials rather than to simplify existing ones.

Table 5–4. Guidelines for Preparing Readable Materials

- Tell the reader only what he or she needs to know
- Use a conversational style and an active voice
- Use short words, sentences, and paragraphs
- Define terms simply at the time that you use them
- Avoid using acronyms and slang
- Avoid abbreviations and contractions

Read the following passage that was designed to inform readers about craniofacial anomalies. The first passage is extracted from *The Genetics of Cleft Lip and Palate; Information for Families* (The Cleft Palate Foundation, 1996) written at college-level readability. Using the guidelines in Table 5–4, it is possible to modify the pamphlet's contents to reflect a lower readability level, appropriate for functionally illiterate adults.

The Cleft Palate Foundation was founded by its parent, the American Cleft Palate-Craniofacial Association, in 1974 to be the public service arm of the professional society. Its primary purpose is *"to enhance the quality of life for individuals with congenital facial deformities and their families through education, research support, and facilitation of family-centered care."*

The Foundation's major activities include the operation of the CLEFTLINE and the dissemination of publications. The CLEFT-LINE is an 800-toll free service providing information and referral to parents of newborns with clefts and other craniofacial anomalies and to affected adults.

This passage poses a number of potential problems for functionally illiterate persons. These include the use of punctuation, difficult-to-read type styles, organization of materials, use of idioms, and inclusion of excessive information.

Punctuation and Organizational Skill

Although the informational brochure is readable and understandable to persons with a reading level of 12th grade or higher, its use of punctuation for conveying information presents significant problems for unskilled readers. Skilled readers know that abstract information is conveyed through the use of punctuation. *Without reading anything,* skilled readers can obtain advance information about written material by glancing at the punctuation before starting to read. Skilled readers know that information contained in quotation marks represents an individual's spoken words. Although capitalization and use of bold font are not strictly punctuation, skilled readers have learned that material presented in bold, all capital, or italicized letters is usually important. In addition, they have the organizational skills necessary to read those sections of the document first if they have no time to read the entire brochure.

Functionally illiterate individuals, by contrast, do not read punctuation or font styles, nor do they generally have the skills necessary to determine which parts of the document are important. They must read the entire document word by word and line by line, an inefficient and time-consuming process.

Use of Idioms

Because unskilled readers interpret information literally, they may be confused by expressions such as, "the Foundation was founded by its *parent*" and "public service *arm* of the professional society." How can a society be a parent? A parent is a *person*, is it not? To an unskilled reader, an arm is a body part, not a division of a professional society. Idioms are especially confusing to persons who speak English as a second language.

Excessive information

Because unskilled readers have poorly developed organizational skills, reading is time consuming. Functionally illiterate individuals want easy access to information that addresses their problem directly. The first paragraph of the information in the brochure is interesting but provides no direct help for a functionally illiterate parent of a child with cleft palate.

Compare the following boxed example to the original passage. Notice that it was written with a conversational style and an active voice. Notice that it includes only pertinent information and that terms are defined at the time that they are used. Clear statements have been substituted. In addition, a complete telephone number has been provided.

Getting Answers to Your Questions

If your baby has a hole in the roof of his or her mouth (a cleft palate), you may have questions. You may wonder why your child was born with this problem. You may want to know what can be done to help your child. We at The Cleft Palate Foundation can help you understand your child's facial problems. We can help you find a doctor to treat your child. If you want to ask some-one about cleft lip or cleft palate, call 1-800-444-5555. *You may call for free.* You will not be charged for this call.

Although the document's contents are now written at a lower grade level, this information can be made even more readable by changing its appearance. Functionally illiterate readers often avoid reading material that looks difficult. Table 5–5 summarizes ways of making printed material look easy to read. We can make the above information look "easy" by choosing a simple, easily legible font such as Geneva. Use *large print* and *wide margins* and *substitute underlining for italics*. The finished document looks like this:

If your baby has a hole in the roof of his or her mouth (a cleft palate), you may have questions. You may wonder why your child was born with this problem. You may want to know what can be done to help your child. We at the Cleft Palate Foundation can help you understand your child's facial problems. We can help you find a doctor to treat your child. If you want to ask someone about cleft lip or cleft palate, call 1-800-444-5555. <u>You may call for free</u>. You will not be charged for this call.

Table 5-5. Making Material Look Readable

- Use large print and wide margins
- Underline for emphasis
- Select a simple, sans serif font
- Don't mix fonts, type sizes, and ink colors

The following passage is extracted from *Feeding an Infant with a Cleft* (Unrich, 1992). This brochure also was prepared by the Cleft Palate Foundation and has a 12th-grade readability level.

If you are concerned that your infant's feedings may be taking too long, discuss your observations with your health care provider to rule out any possibility of formula intolerance, upper respiratory infection, etc., or request a consultation with the feeding consultant on your local cleft palate/craniofacial team.

Before rewriting, try to determine what the main readability problems are. Although it is written in a conversational style and an active voice, there is clearly an organizational problem. This paragraph is only *one sentence long*. The following is an example of the same passage rewritten using several sentences, simplified terminology, and only pertinent information.

Babies with cleft palate often take a long time to feed. If you think your baby is taking too long to finish his bottle tell your doctor. Let your doctor know if your baby falls asleep while feeding. Your doctor may need to adjust your baby's formula. You may need to use a softer nipple. You may need to use a nipple with a larger opening. Ask the doctor to have someone show you the best way to feed your baby.

The rewritten material now has a readability level of approximately Grade 4.5. This passage is written in an active voice, and technical terminology and abbreviations have been removed. It provides only information the patient needs to know and is organized in short, informative sentences. Again, the document could be modified to make it look easy to read.

Modifying Forms

Forms, unlike brochures, usually contain sentence fragments and brief phrases. Like brochures, forms should have a clear purpose and a logical organization, contain only essential information, and appear easy to read. Although forms cannot be evaluated accurately using readability formulas, any form can be made more readable by removing or changing the number of difficult features it contains.

Readability issues are important to remember when designing or revising forms. Forms present an additional level of difficulty for functionally illiterate individuals because they require written responses. Functionally illiterate adults usually have developed coping strategies for concealing problems with reading and writing. These strategies can often be observed when written information is requested from a patient. If your clinic requires patients to complete forms on site, notice who completes the written information. Be alert, but not judgmental, if a patient asks to take a form home or asks a family member to fill out the paperwork. These requests are sometimes, although not always, indicative of an underlying reading problem. Figure 5–1 illustrates a page from a generic case history form. This form can be modified to make it easier to read by using the guidelines summarized in Table 5–6.

At first glance, the form seems readable. The questions require short answers or check marks, and the lists of questions in the medical history section are short. A second look, however, reveals problems of organization, document appearance, terminology, and content.

Organization

Forms, like other written materials, should be logically organized. Case history forms are usually organized chronologically and divided into sections preceded by organizational headers. The sample form contains organizational headers but could be improved by moving the instructions to the beginning of the form.

Central University
Speech and Hearing Clinic
45 Elm Street
Central City, OH 45056

Phone: (616) 523-1234
Fax: (616) 523-1235

CHILD SPEECH-LANGUAGE CASE HISTORY

Child's Name _____ Date _____ BD ____ Age _____
Address _____
Parents' Names _____
Marital Status_____ Occupation _____
Home Phone _____ Work Phone _____
Who referred this child to this clinic? _____
Why was this child referred to this clinic? _____
Name and relationship of person completing form _____
_____

Has this child been seen by an ENT? _____ If yes,
please provide name and address of the doctor _____
_____

Please answer all questions as completely as possible. This information is important for complete evaluation of the problem. All information will be held in confidence and used only in a professional manner.

Medical History
Please indicate the age at which this child experienced any of these conditions:

Rubella   _____   Meningitis   _____
Tonsillectomy   _____   Otitis media   _____
Malnutrition   _____   Seizures   _____

Is there any history of the following in the family? (please check).
☐ Alcoholism   ☐ Child abuse
☐ Hearing loss   ☐ Cleft palate
☐ Speech impairments   ☐ Heart problems
☐ Marijuana use   ☐ Cocaine use

Figure 5–1. Example of a case history form that could be made more readable. Note mixture of fonts, use of abbreviations, medical terminology, and inclusion of incriminating questions.

Table 5-6. Guidelines for Preparing or Modifying Forms

- Use a conversational style and an active voice
- Use short, complete sentences
- Organize the form logically
- Ask only for essential information
- Avoid using abbreviations
- Substitute simple expressions for medical terms
- Use check lists instead of discussion questions
- Save controversial issues for oral interviews
- Keep font and type size consistent
- Remove redundant material

Appearance

Because functionally illiterate readers have difficulty reading abbreviations, words written in all capital letters, fancy fonts, and small print, it is best to avoid using such features. The ease and versatility of word processing programs often encourage users to cross the line from functional to creative when designing forms. Resist the temptation to be visually creative and keep font style and size simple and consistent when writing or revising a form.

Terminology

Medical words are often long and visually daunting to unskilled readers. Use the shortest, most commonly accepted terms to describe medical conditions. In this form, substitute measles for rubella, and earaches for otitis media. In some geographic regions, seizures are often called fits or spells. In order to avoid including misleading terminology such as fits on forms be prepared to orally restate some of the form's contents. Remember that you can discuss the form's information with the patient or patient's family. Intake forms provide guidance, but do not substitute for in-depth oral patient interviews.

Sensitive Content

Keep the form's purpose in mind when deciding what questions to include. Examine the document's contents carefully. Ask yourself, "Why am I asking that question?" and "Am I likely to get an honest answer?" Issues of drug abuse, child abuse, and malnutrition have implications beyond that of readability. Sensitive material or questions with legal implications are probably best explored in a context other than a written form. Keep the form short and save controversial issues for in-depth interview situations.

Confusing Instructions

Because unskilled readers are likely to interpret information literally, instructions must be very clear. "Is there any history of the following in the family? (please check)," could be literally interpreted to mean "ask your family members about health problems." In this case, the instructions mean that the reader should place a check mark beside each condition that occurs in his or her family.

Writing Style

Use short, complete sentences and write in an active voice using a conversational style. For example, change "Who referred this child to this clinic?" to "Who asked you to bring your child to our clinic?" Substitute "Birthday" for "BD," and "throat doctor" for "ENT."

Modifying Legal Documents

Parental consent, release of clinical information, and permission to publish patient photographs require the patient to sign forms that serve as legal documents. Specific material regarding content of photograph release forms is addressed in Chapter 7.

Because legal documents represent binding agreements, they are often written in long sentences, a passive voice, and legal terminology. Legal documents can be made more readable by using the suggestions for modifying forms. In most cases, it is the *content* of the document's material, not the language in which it is written, that is important. Major institutions and businesses often have a legal advisor on staff. If such a professional is available, ask him or her to critique your rewritten legal form for accuracy and completeness of content.

Finally, because legal documents are binding agreements, we must be certain that all patients understand the contents of the forms they are asked to sign. It is good policy to read the document aloud to the patient, pausing after each paragraph, and allowing time for questions. As further insurance against misunderstandings, ask the patient to restate what you said. You can then explain further, if necessary.

SUMMARY

Because the illiteracy rate is high, health care professionals must not assume that patients can read clinical materials and forms. Be alert for patients who may be functionally illiterate and modify clinical materials accordingly. Be prepared to answer questions, clarify material, and take the additional time needed to educate patients. Illiteracy is, after all, a communication problem.

EXPANDING YOUR KNOWLEDGE BASE

The following readings offer detailed information that clinicians may find useful.

Hegde, M. N., & Davis, D. (1995). Working with clients. In *Clinical methods and practicum in speech-language pathology* (2nd ed., pp. 99–142). San Diego, CA: Singular Publishing Group.

Middleton, G. F., & Pannbacker, M. (1997). Speech-language screening and assessment. In *Cleft palate and related disorders* (pp. 113–174). Bisbee, AZ: Imaginart International.

Peterson, H. A., & Marquardt, T. P. (1990). Clinical reporting and record keeping. In *Appraisal and diagnosis of speech and language disorders* (2nd ed., pp. 294–310). Englewood Cliffs, NJ: Prentice Hall.

Pozger, G. D. (1990). *Legal aspects of health care administration* (4th ed.). Gaithersburg, MD: Aspen Publishers.

Roth, F. P., & Worthington, C. K. (1996). Information reporting systems and techniques. In F. P. Roth & C. K. Worthington (Eds.), *Treatment resource manual for speech-language pathology* (pp. 56–83). San Diego, CA: Singular Publishing Group.

Shipley, K. G., & McAfee, J. G. (1998). Reporting assessment findings. In *Assessment in speech-language pathology: A resource manual* (2nd ed., pp. 67–84). San Diego, CA: Singular Publishing Group.

REFERENCES

The Cleft Palate Foundation. (1980). *Information for the teenager born with a cleft lip and/or palate* [Brochure]. Pittsburgh, PA: Author.

The Cleft Palate Foundation. (1996). *The genetics of cleft lip and palate: Information for families* (2nd ed.) [Brochure]. Pittsburgh, PA: Author.

Doak, C. C., Doak, L. G., & Root, K. J. (1985). *Teaching patients with low literacy skills*. Philadelphia: J. B. Lippincott Co.

Frager, A., & Kahn, A. (1988). How useful are elementary school health text-books for teaching about hearing health and protection? *Language, Speech, and Hearing Services in Schools, 19,* 175–181.

Heisel, M., & Larson, G. (1984). Literacy and social milieu: Reading behavior of the black elderly. *Adult Education Quarterly, 34 ,* 63–70.

Kahn, A. & Pannbacker, M. (in press). Readability of educational materials for families and clients with cleft palate. *American Journal of Speech-language Pathology.*

Kelly, L., & Kahn, A. (1991). Illiteracy and hearing loss management: the readability of clinic forms. *Journal of the Academy of Rehabilitative Audiology, 24,* 35–42.

Kelly, L. (1996). The readability of hearing aid brochures. *Journal of Research Audiology, 29,* 41–47.

Laidlaw, J., & Harden, R. (1987). Printed material for patients with heart disease: Are we really educating patients? *Medical Teacher 9,* 201–204.

National Center for Education Statistics. (1993). *Adult Literacy in America* (GPO Stock No. 065-000-00588-3). Washington, DC: Government Printing Office.

Unrich, K. (1992). *Feeding an infant with a cleft* [Brochure]. Pittsburgh, PA: Cleft Palate Foundation.

CHAPTER 6

BUILDING A PROFESSIONAL SUPPORT SYSTEM

As students, future SLPs have access to multidisciplinary learning environments, medical equipment, computer technology, and libraries. More important, they are encouraged to pursue personal avenues of interest, interact directly with medical professionals, and discuss the latest developments in patient care. Although not all speech-language pathology programs meet the above criteria, most offer resources and opportunities that are not readily available to the majority of SLPs working outside a university or medical environment.

The transition from student status to full-time employment is sometimes a challenging one. After graduating and obtaining American Speech-Language and Hearing Association (ASHA) certification, SLPs may feel overwhelmed by employment realities such as caseload size, workspace constraints, insurance reimbursement problems, and lack of funding for the purchase of minimal diagnostic and therapy materials. Students accustomed to attending interdisciplinary conference sessions may be initially dismayed to find themselves serving large numbers of patients with little support from or interaction with other SLPs.

Such working conditions pose a unique set of challenges, not the least of which is insuring that patients receive appropriate diagnosis and treatment. Fortunately, these challenges though difficult, are surmountable. Resources are available locally, nationally, and (thanks to the

Internet) internationally. SLPs who seriously wish to do so can build an effective professional support system, even from remote or poorly funded work settings. Building a support system requires an initial personal investment of time and money and an ongoing commitment to continuing education and professional service. Most SLPs begin creating a support system through the process of networking—meeting and interacting with individuals who have similar career goals and professional interests.

BUILDING PROFESSIONAL RELATIONSHIPS

Networking often begins while individuals are earning professional degrees, particularly during graduate school. Professors, fellow students, and medical professionals at extern placement sites all comprise an initial group of professionals with whom to share ideas, projects, or future plans. Unfortunately, these initial contacts are often disrupted upon graduation, especially if new graduates relocate to settings distant from their educational facility. Along with the challenges of working unassisted for the first time, newly certified SLPs must interact with unfamiliar coworkers while learning their employer's expectations. Many SLPs turn to fellow professionals for assistance in treating difficult patients, making specific diagnoses of unfamiliar conditions, and for general professional support in an unfamiliar work environment. Ideally, such professional support is available from coworkers with advanced therapy skills and experience. Accurate diagnosis and treatment of craniofacial anomalies require a specialized level of expertise, however, and not all facilities will have employees who meet such standards. In such situations, SLPs who want to network with craniofacial specialists must rely on contacts made outside their immediate environment. Craniofacial specialists can be contacted in several ways: through professional organizations, during visits to craniofacial teams, at state or national conventions, and through Internet resources.

Professional Organizations

Many student SLPs receive their first contact with professional organizations when they join the National Student Speech-Language and Hearing Association (NSSLHA); upon graduation, almost all SLPs become members of the American Speech-Language and Hearing Association (ASHA). As the major U.S. professional association for SLPs and audiologists, ASHA provides its members with certification, professional journals and newsletters, an annual convention, continuing education opportunities, and employment information. ASHA also serves as the umbrella organization for a number of focused special interest divisions.

ASHA Special Interest Division 5: Speech Science and Orofacial Disorders (SID 5)

SLPs and audiologists who want to interact with professionals specializing in craniofacial anomalies may begin by joining ASHA Special Interest Division 5 (SID 5). John Riski (1997) described the primary role of SID 5 as fostering partnerships between a number of groups, including clinicians and scientists, school settings and medical settings, and academic settings and clinical settings.

After joining the group, individuals may access the SID 5 List serve and maintain direct E-mail correspondence with other SID 5 members, who are primarily SLPs and audiologists with interest and experience in the fields of speech science and craniofacial anomalies. Members also receive newsletters and updates on research developments, job opportunities, and grant information. As of 1999, efforts continued between SID 5 and the American Cleft Palate-Craniofacial Association (ACPA) to schedule collaborative workshops for public school clinicians.

American Cleft Palate-Craniofacial Association (ACPA)

Although SID 5 is a valuable organization for persons who are interested in craniofacial anomalies, it has a dual focus: speech science and orofacial disorders. Health care professionals who have limited interest in speech science issues may wish to join the American Cleft Palate-Craniofacial Association (ACPA) instead of, or in addition to, SID 5.

The ACPA is an international, nonprofit, multidisciplinary medical society whose members treat and conduct research on birth anomalies of the head and face. As of 1999, the ACPA had more than 2600 members representing over 30 disciplines in 40 countries. Members of the ACPA receive quarterly newsletters containing research updates, information about craniofacial programs and cleft palate teams, grant and funding opportunities, and schedules of upcoming craniofacial conventions and conferences.

SLPs needing specific information about location and composition of craniofacial teams can find this material in the ACPA's *Membership-Team Directory*. The directory contains an alphabetical listing of members of the ACPA, as well as a geographic listing of team members and craniofacial teams. Information about current officers, committees, and editorial boards, as well as copies of the ACPA constitution, by-laws, and code of ethics are included.

The ACPA holds annual scientific meetings and publishes the bi-monthly *Cleft Palate-Craniofacial Journal*. This journal contains articles about clinical activities and research in cleft lip and or cleft palate and craniofacial anomalies. Like ASHA, the ACPA has a Web site (see Table 6–1) for easily accessing information regarding membership, conventions and professional meetings, and officers of the association. It also has a nonprofit public service affiliate, the Cleft Palate Foundation (CPF).

The Cleft Palate Foundation (CPF)

The Cleft Palate Foundation (CPF) was founded by the ACPA in 1973. According to the *1999–2000 ACPA Membership Team Directory*, the CPF's primary purpose is "to optimize care of persons affected by craniofacial anomalies through professional education, stimulation of research, and the promotion of interdisciplinary collaboration and team care." The CPF's toll-free telephone service (see Table 6–1) is available to parents of children with craniofacial anomalies or to adults with craniofacial anomalies. Callers can receive information about support groups, the availability of craniofacial teams, or specific craniofacial anomalies. Approximately 20 fact sheets and brochures about craniofacial anomalies are available free to families (and at cost to professionals). The CPF also provides annual research grants to researchers.

AboutFace

Although the CPF is an excellent resource for SLPs, its major focus is on diagnosing and treating patients with *congenital* craniofacial anomalies. Patients who have acquired craniofacial anomalies as a result of accident or disease may need information or support from an organization with a broader focus. AboutFace is one such organization.

Since 1985, AboutFace has provided information, support, and education to persons with facial differences and their families. AboutFace was founded in Canada, and in 1991 a chapter was formed in the United States. AboutFace publishes professional publications and an international newsletter. It also offers a Web site and a network of members who can provide emotional support to persons with facial anomalies. Unlike the ACPA, AboutFace does not offer information on treatment options or medical referrals. Because it emphasizes parent and family support systems, and because it addresses acquired as well as congenital facial anomaly issues, AboutFace is a useful broad-spectrum support organization.

Organizations for Specific Craniofacial Problems

Some craniofacial conditions occur only rarely, and persons with those conditions are infrequently encountered by SLPs and the general population. Nationally, however, persons having these conditions may be numerous enough to encourage the formation of national and local support groups. Although the average SLP working outside a medical setting is unlikely to encounter a child with Treacher Collins syndrome, for example, it is important to be aware of specific support groups for such rare disorders in case such an unlikely event occurs. One of the best, most comprehensive Web sites listing support groups for persons with specific craniofacial anomalies is the Genetic/Rare Conditions Support Groups & Information Web site at [http://www.kumc.edu/gec/support]. This and other useful Web sites are described later in this chapter.

In summary, craniofacially focused professional organizations can provide SLPs with continuing education opportunities, research funds, and employment opportunities. Most important, membership in such organizations brings the opportunity to interact with professionals who specialize in diagnosing and treating craniofacial anomalies. The negative aspects of belonging to such organizations are minor and are largely financial. Table 6–1 compares the major professional support organizations available to SLPs in the United States. Notice that annual dues for active membership are sometimes significant. Many SLPs pay dues, licensure, and certification fees to state and regional professional organizations, as well as to ASHA, and additional membership in one or more specialized organizations represents further financial commitment. Nonetheless, specialized memberships can provide specific educational opportunities and professional contacts that may be found nowhere else. Many SLPs view these expenses as a small investment for a very large professional return.

Site Visits to Craniofacial Teams

Patients with craniofacial anomalies often benefit from a multidisciplinary approach to diagnosis and treatment, especially if problems with velopharyngeal competence are present. Despite the fact that there is currently little scientific evidence about efficacy (Shprintzen, 1995), team treatment is often perceived to be more accurate, economical, and convenient than treatment provided locally in a nonteam setting. At the least, patients and their families should be aware of all available options before selecting a treatment program. SLPs can assist in the selection process by visiting regional craniofacial teams, meeting team members,

Table 6–1. Comparison of Professional Craniofacial Organizations

Organization	Annual Membership Fee	Web site/Telephone/ E-mail
AboutFace Canada 99 Crowns Lane, 4th Floor Toronto, Ontario M6H 3M8 Canada	None; donations encouraged	www.interlog.com/~abtface/ 1-800-665-FACE E-mail address available on Web site
AboutFace USA P.O. Box 93 Limekiln, PA 19535		
American Cleft Palate-Craniofacial Association 104 South Estes Dr. Suite 204 Chapel Hill, NC 27514	Student Member: $65.00 no initial entrance fee Active, Associate, or International Member: $125.00; initial entrance fee: $25.00	www.cleft.com (919) 933-9044 E-mail address available on Web site
American Speech-Language and Hearing Association 10801 Rockville Pike Rockville, MD 20852	Active Member: $174.00; $25.00 for special interest division memberships	www.asha.org (888) 321-ASHA
Cleft Palate Foundation 104 South Estes Dr. Suite 204 Chapel Hill, NC 27514	None; nonprofit. Donations encouraged	www.cleft.com/cpf.htm (919) 933-9044

and learning something about each team's methods of operation and their referral and treatment policies.

As of 1999, the number of craniofacial teams within each U.S. state ranged from a low of one team in states such as Delaware, New Hampshire, and New Mexico, to a high of 23 teams in the state of California. Numbers do not always reflect team accessibility. For example, although the small state of Rhode Island has only one craniofacial team it is located near several more teams in surrounding states. On the other hand, Alaska, a large, geographically remote state with a comparatively small population has only two such teams.

SLPs can learn about state or regional craniofacial teams by reading descriptive information in the *ACPA Membership Team Directory*. The directory publishes team locations, specific contact information, and names and addresses of contact persons who are members of the ACPA. It also contains detailed team descriptions, including information such as the number of team meetings per calendar year; the number of new patients seen per year; the number of treatment and follow-up procedures performed; and a breakdown of specific types of treatments performed.

Such basic information provides a starting point for understanding local and regional team services, but it leaves questions like quality of care and team interaction issues unanswered. SLPs who want to know more about quality and effectiveness of craniofacial teams before making patient referrals to those teams can arrange a site visit to observe the team in action.

Personal site visits can be arranged by contacting the craniofacial team's coordinator. Most teams are accustomed to hosting visiting observers. Because some teams are affiliated with medical schools and require student interns to visit or participate in team functions, visitation space may be limited. Always plan site visits well in advance and expect last minute changes to occur. SLPs who are providing therapy to a patient who is under team care may arrange to accompany their patient on a trip to the craniofacial team if plans are made in advance. Because organization and length of team meetings vary from team to team, it is best to ask the team's policy when scheduling a site visit.

Site visits can serve several purposes including forming new professional relationships, learning the team's referral and treatment policies, obtaining specific diagnostic information about patients undergoing treatment, discovering sources of funding for patients with special financial needs, and understanding the treatment options provided by a particular team. Whenever possible, SLPs should visit several craniofacial teams to compare patient services and quality of care and to personally meet as many interdisciplinary professionals as possible. Craniofacial team members can become valuable resources in an SLP's professional network.

Site visits, although valuable in the long term, initially can be costly and time consuming. A visit to a craniofacial team may require from 1 to 3 days, depending on location. Although some employers consider site visits continuing education, not all will understand, finance, or approve of such an investment of time away from work. In such cases, SLPs have the choice of using personal vacation or leave time to complete site visits or of attempting to meet craniofacial team members in some other setting.

Conventions

State and national conventions provide good forums for making professional contacts while simultaneously contributing to continuing education. Because continuing education is desirable, and often necessary to obtain or renew state certification, most employers encourage SLPs to pursue continuing education opportunities. Many employers offer employees at least one annual opportunity to attend state or national conventions. Professional meetings are logical places to complete continuing education requirements, and they also provide ideal opportunities for meeting craniofacial experts and members of craniofacial teams.

Selecting the most appropriate convention or conventions to attend depends largely on the SLP's purpose. SLPs who want to obtain current information about diagnosis and treatment of craniofacial anomalies may choose from workshops offered at state conventions or national scientific meetings. Organizations such as ASHA, ACPA, or The American Academy of Audiology (AAA) usually include educational craniofacial material in convention programs. In addition, both ASHA and ACPA periodically sponsor special state or regional workshops on genetic and craniofacial issues.

SLPs who attend professional meetings with the goal of contacting members of craniofacial teams would do well to attend the ACPA Annual Meeting. Because this meeting is a multidisciplinary, international convention, it is more likely to attract a variety of craniofacial team members than is a specific convention organized for SLPs, audiologists, nurses, or other members of the health care professions.

In addition to providing an opportunity to meet members of one or several craniofacial teams, SLPs can learn something about the professional goals and expertise of team members by carefully reviewing the convention program in advance. Often team members not only attend the convention, but make professional presentations as well. Attending such presentations offers a good opportunity to access the expertise of team members as they describe research projects or teach diagnostic or therapy techniques.

Internet Resources

Although attending professional meetings allows SLPs to discuss current issues and form professional relationships, they cannot entirely take the place of day-to-day interaction with an expert in craniofacial diagnosis and treatment. When an SLP needs immediate answers to questions about referral sources, therapy methods, parent support groups, and continuing education, it is sometimes more effective to use computer resources. SLPs who have computer access sometimes find that professional networking is as convenient as logging on to the Internet.

Although computer access is widespread, it is by no means universal. Budget constraints can cause even the most progressive hospitals, schools, and clinics to make stringent decisions regarding purchase and use of computer technology. SLPs who cannot log on to the Internet at their work setting may have to rely on a home personal computer or on computers available at a local public library. In any event, Internet resources can connect SLPs to an abundant variety of craniofacial resources efficiently, easily, and affordably. New Internet users may be daunted by the sheer abundance of available information. The tasks of finding accurate, reliable, ethical sources of information about a specific topic may at first seem too time consuming to be worth the effort. This task can be simplified by becoming familiar with basic Internet operation and by accessing reliable Web sites specifically maintained to provide information about craniofacial anomalies.

It is beyond the scope of this textbook to teach basic computer skills and Internet operation. Novice Internet users who want basic information about Internet safety and operation, E-mail, list serves, Web page construction, or similar issues should consult references such as *Harley Hahn Teaches the Internet* (Hahn, 1999), *Building Learning Communities in Cyberspace* (Pallof & Pratt, 1999), and similar resource materials. With practice, finding and exchanging information on the Internet becomes faster and easier. Accessing reliable Web sites is one way to begin.

Three Web Sites

There are thousands of specific Web sites describing craniofacial organizations, therapy techniques, support organizations, and specific craniofacial anomalies. Most have links to similar Web sites, and many provide names and contact information of persons who are "experts" on various craniofacial anomalies. It is important to remember that information on the Internet, unlike information found in most textbooks and professional journals, does not have to undergo an editorial review process before being published. In other words, information found on the Internet may represent the opinion of the site's creator and may or may not be accurate or current. Although it is tempting to believe that information on a Web site is accurate, valid, and endorsed by a particular group or agency, the fact is that anyone can construct a Web site and place it on the Internet. Web sites provide a quick source for reference material, but it is the user's responsibility to determine whether or not the reference material is valid. Despite the prevalence of inaccurate or actively fraudulent Web sites, reliable craniofacial resource information is available on the Internet. In addition to the Web sites of ASHA, ACPA, and AboutFace, the following three sources are particularly useful: Online Mendelian Inheritance in Man; Genetic/Rare Conditions Support Groups and Information; and The Boys Town Research Registry for Hereditary Hearing Loss.

Online Mendelian Inheritance in Man (OMIM)

OMIM is a database catalog of genetic disorders. It was developed and edited at Johns Hopkins by Dr. Victor McKusick and colleagues and was placed on the Internet by the National Center for Biotechnology Information. Because it was developed for use by physicians and genetic researchers, this site is recommended for persons who want advanced scientific information. The site has useful links to MEDLINE articles and to images contained in an archive at the Neonatology page on the Web site. OMIM at [http://www3.ncbi.nlm.nih.gov/omim/] is an excellent source of advanced material about genes and genetic disorders.

Genetic/Rare Conditions Support Groups and Information

Developed by the University of Kansas Medical Center, this Web site serves professionals who want information on rare conditions or birth defects. This site provides links to other sites describing specific genetic and rare conditions. Additional links connect the user to specific national and international support organizations and to government consumer health information. Information for locating genetic counselors and finding support for siblings of children with genetic and or rare conditions is also included. There are also links to translation services to languages including Spanish, German, French, Russian, Vietnamese, and sign language. This site [http://www.kumc.edu/gec/support] is updated and verified regularly and is an excellent source of information for the general public, as well as for professionals in search of specific information for rare conditions.

The Boys Town Research Registry for Hereditary Hearing Loss

Because many craniofacial anomalies involve hearing loss and hereditary forms of deafness, it is important to have reliable sources of information about hearing loss. The Boys Town Research Registry is one such source. This Web site is designed to foster partnerships between families, clinicians, and researchers who are interested in hereditary hearing loss. The Registry collects information from individuals who wish to participate in hearing-loss-related research. It also provides information about hearing loss to professionals and families and uses this information to match families to specific research projects. This site [http://www.boystown. org/deafgene.reg/] provides links to fact sheets on specific topics such as Fundamentals of Hearing, Autism and Deafness: A Psychologist's Perspective, Ten Syndromes Most Commonly Associated With Hearing Impairment, and Waardenburg syndrome. It also has links to current research projects and surveys. This is an excellent source of information for members of the general public, as well as professional researchers.

List Serves

Although each of the above Web sites provides specific names, locations, and E-mail addresses for individuals connected with each site, they are not primarily designed to encourage professional on-line discussions. Such exchanges are better conducted through a list serve. A list serve is a mailing list that allows a group of people to interact with one another through E-mail. It differs from ordinary E-mail in that a message sent to a list serve is delivered to all members of that list serve. Although list serves allow members to ask questions of everyone, only those persons with useful information or interest in the subject generally respond. List serves allow novices to interact with advanced professionals, and they do so in a non-threatening, efficient manner. Many organizations form List serves so that their members can communicate with one another on-line on a convenient, as-needed basis.

CLEFTSERVE

The ACPA provides its members with CLEFTSERVE, a List serve created by the ACPA and the University of Iowa Department of Otolaryngology—Head and Neck Surgery. This list serve is restricted to use by ACPA members only. After subscribing to CLEFTSERVE, ACPA members can exchange information with, and ask questions of, leading national and international experts in the disciplines associated with craniofacial care and research. CLEFTSERVE is particularly useful because it is an interdisciplinary, international list serve, and because its use is restricted to professionals interested in craniofacial issues. Persons using CLEFTSERVE can exchange information with surgeons, nurses, audiologists, SLPs, pediatricians, orthodontists, or anyone who is a member of the ACPA. CLEFTSERVE is an extremely valuable tool for novices and experts alike.

SUMMARY

Developing professional relationships is personally, educationally, and professionally rewarding. Although establishing a professional support system takes time, effort, and sometimes a financial investment, with the development of Internet resources, the problems associated with working in remote locations are lessened. Individuals who have an interest in craniofacial anomalies have a variety of options for continuing their education and for meeting professionals with similar interests. These options include joining and participating in state and national professional organizations planning site visits to meet members of craniofacial teams attending craniofacial conferences and workshops and interacting with experts via the Internet and list serves. Making and maintaining professional relationships is an exciting and rewarding experience that benefits the professional—and ultimately the persons that professional serves.

REFERENCES

American Cleft Palate-Craniofacial Association. 1999–2000 *Membership-Team Directory*. Chapel Hill, NC: J. B. Moon.

Hahn, H. (1999). *Harley Hahn teaches the Internet*. Indianapolis, IN: Que Corporation.

Palloff, R. & Pratt, K. (1999). *Building Learning Communities in Cyberspace*. San Francisco, CA: Jossey-Bass Publishers.

Riski, J. (1997). Coordinator's corner. *Special Interest Division 5: Speech Science and Orofacial Disorders Newsletter, 7*, 1–2.

Shprintzen, R. J. (1995). A new perspective on clefting. In R. J. Shprintzen & J. Bardach (Eds.), *Cleft palate speech management* (pp. 1–15). St. Louis, MO: C.V. Mosby.

CHAPTER 7

PHOTODOCUMENTING YOUR OBSERVATIONS

Most SLPs include detailed written descriptions of their patients' communication problems as part of case history reports. Occasionally, clinical reports of patients with unusually challenging communication disorders contain supplementary video or audiotaped speech, voice, and language samples. Historically, however, SLPs working in nonmedical settings have not routinely used 35 mm photographs to enhance written descriptions. On the other hand, craniofacial team members routinely use photography for diagnostic and comparative purposes.

It is not surprising that photography is frequently used in hospitals and clinics because these facilities often employ full time medical photographers and maintain on-site photographic studios. Some research centers use both traditional photography and computer technology for patient photography and for production and archival storage of educational materials. Although optimal photographic conditions are enviable, they are not necessary for the production of high-quality photographic images. This chapter explains the purposes and advantages of taking 35 mm photographs, considerations for selecting basic equipment, tips for taking accurate patient photographs, and ethical and legal photographic considerations. Photography is a clinical skill that, as with all skills, improves with practice. Because photographs can contribute valuable visual information to the diagnosis and treatment of patients with craniofacial anomalies, it is a skill worth learning and perfecting.

ADVANTAGES OF PHOTODOCUMENTATION

Some SLPs question the necessity of using medical photography in routine clinical practice because of the additional time, skill, and expense the process entails. Incorporating medical photography into the repertoire of clinical skills often requires novice photographers to learn to use unfamiliar equipment. Proficient photographers often must acquire a different mind set regarding the purpose and technique of clinical photography. Individuals accustomed to taking photographs of family events or scenic places must understand the differences between informal photography and medical photography.

Medical photography differs from informal photography in purpose and technique. Informal photographs are usually taken for pleasure, with the general goal of recording persons or events in the most favorable and attractive way. Medical photography, however, is a formal process requiring the written consent of the person photographed. The goal of medical photography is to visually record a patient's appearance as *accurately* as possible under consistent and measurable photographic conditions. The resulting photographs can be used for a variety of purposes, including identifying patients, diagnosing craniofacial syndromes, comparing longitudinal changes, and preparing educational materials.

Patient Identification

Although the chance that a given work setting will experience disaster conditions is small, the risk of living in what is sometimes a dangerous and litigious society suggests that SLPs do their part to ensure their patients' safety. Risks exist in the safest environments. For example, children and neurologically impaired adults occasionally stray from health care facilities, parents undergoing marital discord sometimes deliberately remove their children from schools and into hiding, criminals occasionally abduct children from public places, and natural disasters occasionally occur. During such unlikely events, current photographs can be invaluable in locating and identifying missing or injured patients. Some work settings require that current photographs be part of every patient's clinical file. This is good policy, as well as good common sense. Visual records are extremely helpful in emergency situations.

Diagnosis of Syndromes

The protocols for visual observation previously described in this textbook can be readily adapted to photographic observation. Photographs taken from anterior, posterior, profile, and superior viewpoints may be used to identify or confirm the presence of unusual craniofacial features. Whole body photographs provide information about height, body proportions, and symmetry. Sometimes unusual facial features overlooked during live observations become immediately apparent in photographs. Although additional observations must be made before syndromes can be positively identified, accurate medical photographs are an important part of the initial diagnostic process.

Observing Longitudinal Changes

In a sense, family photographs reflect longitudinal, age-related changes in the appearance of family members. Many families have photographic records spanning more than a century, allowing observation of physical changes in past as well as present generations of family members. Medical photography also systematically records changes produced by normal growth and aging, as well as those produced by surgical or medical procedures. Craniofacial teams routinely use 35 mm photographs, cephalometric radiography, and CT scans to record changes in the cranial base, dentition, and facial bones. These procedures are performed consistently so that changes can be measured and future changes can be predicted based on photographic comparisons.

Although the average SLP in a nonmedical setting may have little need to record or predict longitudinal changes, such changes do occur and constitute an important part of the patient's clinical record. Events as "minor" as normal loss of the deciduous middle incisors or reconfiguration of dentition with orthodontic appliances can significantly affect speech production. Keeping annual or semi-annual photographic records can assist in tracking the progress of age-related events and medical procedures.

Preparing Professional Educational Materials

Students and newly certified SLPs often think in terms of *acquiring* rather than *providing* continuing education. This is understandable at the outset of a career because at that time most individuals have limited professional expertise to share. Over time, professional goals often expand to include providing continuing education to members of the general community and to fellow professionals. Photographs are an excellent way to record, preserve, and illustrate clinical events for educational presentations. High-quality archivally preserved photographs are timeless and remain to illustrate professional presentations decades after they were initially taken. Archival storage has become easier now that photographs can be scanned and stored digitally on disk, CD-ROM, or other media. SLPs who plan to become professional educators can increase their chances for success by maintaining visual records of interesting patients.

SELECTING PHOTOGRAPHIC EQUIPMENT

The basic equipment needed for medical photography includes a camera body, a camera lens, film, and an appropriate light source—usually an electronic flash attachment. Additional equipment such as tripods, filters, macro brackets, and computer scanners are desirable but not essential to the production of good photographs.

The most basic piece of equipment is the camera. Most of this chapter describes photographic techniques using 35 mm single lens reflex (SLR) cameras. Other types of cameras are suitable for medical photography, and these are described below.

Cameras

Before purchasing an expensive array of photographic equipment, would-be photographers need to assess personal needs and long-term career goals. Although 35 mm SLR photography is a versatile and affordable way to record patient information, it is not the only available photographic method, nor is it necessarily the best choice for novice photographers. Other camera types include Polaroids that develop film instantly, convenient one-time use disposables, user-friendly point and shoot models, and high-tech digital cameras that do not use film at all but record the image on disk or other media. Although all these cameras are capable of making acceptable photographic images, not all are ideal for medical photography. Table 7–1 compares the types of cameras most SLPs are likely to find useful and affordable. Other specialized cameras are available, but these are usually expensive and designed for professional photographers.

Excellent 35 mm SLR cameras are produced by all major camera manufacturers; finding high-quality equipment is seldom a problem. Instead, selection of the "best" camera depends on factors such as the purpose of the photography; the ease of operation; initial cost and upkeep expenses; availability of film, batteries, and developing services; preference for particular special features; and the expertise of the camera operator. SLPs who have little expertise in photography and no desire to keep long-term visual records of patients will probably be satisfied with the results of Polaroid or point-and-shoot cameras. On the other hand, SLPs who conduct large screenings of young children, often

Table 7-1. Comparison of Camera Types

Polaroid Cameras

Advantages

- Easily operated, produce instant photographic images
- Good choice for taking initial photographs of rare or unusual conditions, useful when photographic results must be immediately observed
- Very affordable depending on model
- Best choice for occasional use by novice photographers, little skill required to produce acceptable photographs

Disadvantages

- Price per photo comparatively expensive; not the most economical choice for taking large quantities of photographs.

One-Time Use 35mm Point-and-Shoot Cameras

Advantages

- Useful for taking patient identification photographs and general informal photography
- Cost effective if used occasionally
- Easily operated, instructions are written on the camera
- Cost limited to initial purchase of camera and film processing; no maintenance or operating cost
- Environmentally friendly, camera materials can be recycled
- Cameras are small, light, easily transportable, and readily obtained throughout the United States and Canada
- Several models are available, including 35 mm or Advanced Photo System cameras that provide choices of print shapes
- Good choice for photographers with some understanding of photography; matching correct version of camera to photographic purpose is essential

Disadvantages

- Manual operation; film, battery, and sometimes flash are built in; need for flash must be determined by photographer
- Not a good economic choice for long term frequent use, or for scientific photography
- Resulting photographic images are of good, but not medically professional, quality

35 mm Point and Shoot Cameras

Advantages

- Good choice for patient identification photographs, informal photography, and in-field medical photography
- Wide range of choice, price, and quality of camera

(continued)

Table 7–1. *(continued)*

- Photographic quality of expensive, full-featured models is comparable to 35 mm SLR cameras

- Best choice for novice photographers who want to learn photography on a good-quality camera; good choice for experienced photographers who want quality, ease of operation, and versatility of equipment without investing in a 35 mm SLR system

Disadvantages

- Some camera models require special lithium batteries; these may be difficult to find in remote areas or foreign countries

- Not a good choice if large numbers of photographs must be taken at one time, especially if camera battery is low

- As batteries lose power, the camera's ability to recharge between shots is reduced; photography takes longer under these conditions

- Basic operation is easy, but selecting from a wide variety of photographic options can initially confuse novice photographers

Advanced Photo System (APS) Point and Shoot Cameras

Advantages

- Same advantages as 35 mm point-and-shoot cameras described above

- Camera is smaller then 35 mm point-and-shoot cameras; film is smaller than 35 mm

- Film loading is simple

- Camera allows a shot-by-shot choice of three different print sizes

- Processed film comes with an index print (all images from a roll of film on a single sheet) for easy reference to negatives

- Negatives are safely stored in the APS original cassette

- APS film scanners can easily convert APS film into digital files

- Good choice for novice photographer with a serious, long-term interest in photography and for advanced photographers who like versatility of print size and computer features

Disadvantages

- Does not have wide array of interchangeable lenses available with 35 mm SLR cameras

35 mm Single Lens Reflex (SLR) Cameras

Advantages

- Extremely versatile cameras; most SLRs allow users to choose between fully automatic point-and-shoot modes or fully manual operation

- Large selection of interchangeable lenses in a variety of focal lengths are available for use with SLR camera body

(continued)

Table 7–1. *(continued)*

- Most models have both autofocus and manual focus features
- Wide variety of flash attachments and freedom to move those attachments from typical top of camera placement
- Many have special features such as mirror prelock, through the lens flash exposure, data imprinting, computer interfaces, and close-up accessories for special types of photography
- Allow users to photograph a wide variety of situations, to shoot fast-action sequences, and to photograph in the dark
- Photographic quality is excellent.
- Well cared for, high-quality, SLR cameras can perform well for decades
- SLR cameras are excellent for patient photography as well as scenic, portrait, informal, and macro photography
- SLR cameras are best for serious photographers who are willing to invest time learning how to operate them and who are willing to make a sometimes substantial investment in high-quality lenses and accessories

Disadvantages

- High quality SLR cameras are moderately to very expensive; costs of special lenses, accessories, and batteries can significantly add to the initial cost of the camera
- Most SLR cameras are heavy and are best transported in a protected camera bag; cameras and accessories are attractive to thieves

Digital Point and Shoot

Advantages

- Good choice if images are to be viewed on computer monitors or transmitted via E-mail
- Photographic images are captured by a light-sensing computer chip; images are stored as digital files
- Digital images can be downloaded directly to a computer
- Computer images can be retouched or changed with appropriate software
- Images can be E-mailed or printed out
- Good choice for serious computer users who want to transmit images through E-mail or place them on Web sites
- Good choice for advanced photographers who want to retouch, change, or otherwise manipulate photographic images using a home photo shop computer system

Disadvantages

- Printed out images may fade or run, especially if exposed to direct sunlight or moisture.
- Extensive equipment (e.g., computers, special software, and scanners) are necessary to achieve best results with digital images

(continued)

Table 7–1. *(continued)*

- High-resolution digital cameras can be very expensive; although technology is improving, less expensive versions do not produce photographic images comparable to those produced by 35 mm SLR or APS cameras

- Maintenance costs of equipment (e.g., camera, computer, software, and scanners) can drive up the price of this photography system

- Computer knowledge is necessary to get the most from digital cameras and peripherals

- Currently, high-quality 35 mm photographs can be scanned into a computer to produce digital images equivalent or superior to those produced by low to moderately priced digital cameras

see patients with craniofacial anomalies, and have access to state-of-the art computer systems would do well to invest in a high-quality digital camera and to learn to use it effectively.

Camera Lenses

One advantage of 35 mm SLR cameras is that they allow the photographer to use a variety of special purpose, interchangeable camera lenses. First-time SLR camera buyers are sometimes surprised to find that they can purchase only a camera body, with no lens at all. This is an advantage to the professional photographer who needs at least two loaded camera bodies to photograph situations such as weddings and public events. Two cameras also provide photographers with back-up equipment in case of camera malfunction. For most photographers, however, one camera body will suffice.

SLR cameras are often sold with a standard 50 mm lens that is adequate for multipurpose amateur photographic situations including landscape photography, sports events, and family gatherings. This medium-priced, multipurpose lens is a good one for the general photographer but is not the optimum lens for medical photography. Individuals on limited budgets may choose not to buy the basic 50 mm lens and purchase a special-purpose lens instead.

Photographing craniofacial anomalies requires a lens that can both accurately reproduce the patient's appearance in a full-body photograph as well as reproduce individual facial features without distorting the photographic image. These qualities can be found in a *macro lens,* a special lens designed to photograph small objects. All major SLR manufacturers offer macro lenses in a variety of price ranges. The best macro lenses have excellent optics and are expensive, generally costing between $400.00 and $500.00 (1999 prices). Some macro lenses have a range of focal lengths (90 to 105 mm), for example, and the focal lengths may vary slightly among manufacturers (100 mm Canon macro versus 101 mm Nikon, for example). A high-quality macro lens is a lifetime investment. Although cheaper versions of macro lenses are tempting, the loss of optical quality will be noticeable in photographs. Remember that the goal of medical photography is to accurately record craniofacial anomalies not to create craniofacial anomalies where none exist.

Because noticeable differences in craniofacial appearance can be created by photographing with several different camera lenses, it is important to use a lens that reproduces features accurately. Notice the difference in craniofacial appearance of the young woman in Figure 7–1. Figure 7–1A was taken with a standard 50 mm lens designed for multi-purpose photography and produced an accurate but not close-up view of the patient's facial features. Figure 7–1B was taken with a 28 mm wide-angle lens, a lens designed for taking panoramic views of scenic places. This lens creates visible distortion if used for patient or portrait photography. Figure 7–1C was taken with a 100 mm macro lens and reproduces the patient's facial features accurately.

Macro lenses are also excellent for portrait photography, making them ideal for taking the two types of photographs most needed for recording craniofacial anomalies: whole body and individual features. Purchasing a new SLR camera and macro lens is an expensive initial investment, but one that will repay the SLP in quality and accuracy of resulting photographs. Current editions of photography magazines routinely contain descriptions of the latest cameras and peripheral equipment. Clinicians who are interested in creating a camera system suitable for taking medical photographs would do well to consult articles by Fann (1998a, 1998b, and 1998c) that provide detailed descriptions of camera, lighting, film, and studio selection.

Film

As with cameras, finding high-quality film is easy; making an appropriate selection from the vast array of available film is more difficult. Knowing the photographic purpose can help narrow the choice of film considerably. Specialized film is available for such variable photographic purposes as surveillance work, glamour photography, baby photography, photojournalism, weddings, and sports photography to name only a few. Film is also available in very short rolls containing only a few exposures and in very long rolls for in-studio loading by commercial photographers.

Before selecting a type of film, the photographer must decide whether the image should be black-and-white or color; what form the final image will take (e.g., print, slide, or scanned); how large the ultimate photograph will be; and what the lighting conditions will be during photography.

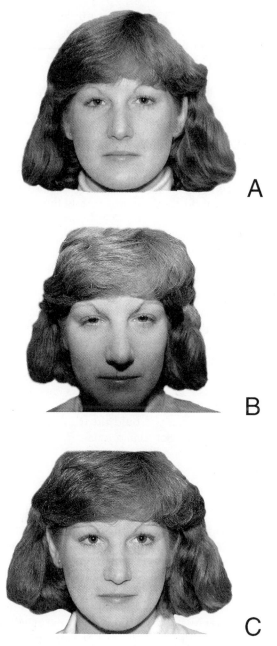

Figure 7–1. Craniofacial appearance of a woman using different camera lenses. Figure 7-1a shows results of photography with 50 mm lens; Figure 7-1b shows photograph taken with 28 mm wide-angle lens; Figure 7-1c shows craniofacial appearance when taken with 100 mm macro lens.

Black and White or Color?

Portrait and scenic photographers must make critical decisions regarding the use of black-and-white or color film, in order to achieve the desired mood in the final photograph. SLPs, on the other hand, have an easier choice when selecting film for photographing patients with craniofacial anomalies.

Because skin, hair, and eye color are significant for diagnosing a number of genetic syndromes, color photographs are generally more useful than are black-and-white images. Color photographs can be also be converted to black-and-white images if necessary. Because *accurate* color reproduction is extremely important, selecting the correct color film is essential.

Currently, there are more than 120 types of 35 mm color film on the market. In addition, film manufacturers constantly discontinue, upgrade, and create new types of film. Because consistency is important in longitudinal photographic studies, it is wise to select a classic film from a major manufacturer. Even this policy may not guarantee film consistency over the years, because even classic films are improved from time to time. The resulting changes are likely to be for the better, however, and are unlikely to produce major noticeable effects on the appearance of photographs in longitudinal studies.

Before purchasing film, it is helpful to compare the features of film types that are currently available. Photography magazines print annual or semiannual buyer's guide issues containing comparative evaluations of photographic equipment, films, and photofinishing services. Reviewing current film evaluations can help narrow film choices to two or three selections. In particular, notice how different brands of film are rated in terms of speed, grain, accuracy of color reproduction, and price.

Speed

Film *speed* describes the film's sensitivity to light. Film speed is expressed as an ISO (International Standards Organization) number that is printed on the film's packaging. Numbers range from very slow ISO 25 to very fast ISO 3200.

Films with very high ISO numbers are best for special photographic situations such as surveillance work, sports events, fashion shows, industrial photography, and news events where ambient light is low and action is high. Photographs taken with very high speed film will be noticeably grainy, particularly when enlarged. Color resolution, contrast, and sharpness are usually reduced. For this reason, high speed film is not the best choice for photographing patients with craniofacial anomalies, particularly if those photographs are going to be enlarged for publication or educational purposes.

Films with very low ISO numbers, by contrast, produce high-resolution, low-grained photographs. Very low speed films require lots of light in order to perform optimally. This is not a problem when electronic flash is used, but it is a concern when photographing with only ambient light. Usually, a low- to medium-speed film such as ISO 100 will provide excellent color, contrast, sharpness, and grain. If photographs are to be enlarged beyond 8 × 10, then an ISO of 50 or lower is desirable, but not essential.

Grain

Photographic images are formed by tiny groups of silver crystals that appear during the developing process. *Grain* describes the appearance of a photograph in terms of the number of individual particles that are visible in the photograph. Often, high speed film produces grainy photographs, especially if the photograph is enlarged. Because grainy photographic images may appear coarse, with blurred edges, selection of a fine-grained film is important. Low- to medium-speed films usually provide very fine grained-images and are recommended for medical photography. Slide films seldom show graininess, even when projected, so film speed is less critical when selecting slide film.

Accuracy of Color Reproduction

Different types of film "see" colors differently, and they do not always see color in the same way the human eye perceives it. When photographing patients for the purpose of diagnosing craniofacial anomalies and assessing general health, it is important to select a film that reproduces color (particularly skin color) as closely as possible to the way the human eye perceives it. Three features are important to accurate color reproduction: resolution, contrast, and color saturation.

Resolution is the ability of film to record fine detail, for example, the striations in the iris of the human eye. Resolution is often expressed as lines per millimeter (l/mm). Some films include resolution numbers on the film packaging. Films with high resolution numbers generally produce sharp photographs with excellent detail.

Contrast, as the term implies, describes the ability to distinguish between adjacent tones in a photograph. Each type of film records a particular range of tones. *High-contrast* film is designed to record a shorter range of tones, but to provide a greater distinction between darker and lighter tones. *Low-contrast* film records a greater range of tones, but the difference between those tones is less visible to the human eye. Contrast varies not only with speed of film, but with film manufacturer. Read descriptions of film ratings carefully and select a low- to medium-speed film that is rated high in contrast.

Color saturation describes the film's ability to record the color of an object at the same intensity on film that it appears in reality. Some films are specifically designed to enhance intensity, making the object more dramatic looking than it actually appears in life. Because medical photography seeks to record appearance in the most *realistic* fashion, color-enhancing films are generally not desirable for clinical photography.

Price

Film cost varies considerably depending on film type, manufacturer's suggestions, place of purchase, and purpose for which the film is designed. Photographic magazines and discount houses often offer "bargain rates" and volume discounts. These "bargains" may offer real value or may be a way of reducing inventory of outdated film, unusual brands of film that require special (and costly) processing, or discontinued types of film. Most nonprofessional photographers can find better, consistent prices by shopping at nationally known discount stores or in local camera dealerships. Film clubs offered by local photo finishers (stores specializing in developing and enlarging film) often give customers substantial discounts on major brand film. When price and film quality are important considerations, it is often less costly in the long run to purchase film from a local, reliable source of major brand films.

After narrowing the choice of film to two or three most suitable to the photographic purpose, it is wise to test the films by photographing the same subject under the same conditions and comparing the resulting photographs or slides. Ideally, photographs should have pleasing sharpness and accurate color reproduction, with little or no visible grain when the image is enlarged.

As with cameras, film choice is also a matter of personal preference. If longitudinal photographic comparisons are to be made, consistency of film type is important. Once a film type is selected, the photographer should continue to use that type of film to photograph the same subject as long as that film is available.

Form and Size of Photograph

Film selection also depends on the desired form and size of the photographic image. Film may be reproduced as 35 mm slides, prints of a variety of sizes, or scanned computer images. Knowing the photographic purpose makes selecting a form easier.

35 mm Slide Film

Slide film is often the film of choice for professional educators who use transparencies for illustrating conference presentations. Slide film is reproduced as transparencies that are mounted in a plastic or cardboard frame and can be projected onto a viewing screen. Transparencies are versatile in that they can be easily converted into prints and computer images. Transparencies are also visually forgiving and seldom show graininess when projected onto a viewing screen. Slide film is versatile, cost effective, and a good choice for professional education, as well as patient photodocumentation purposes.

Print Film

Print film produces photographic images on paper; these images can be enlarged. Because paper contains chemicals and comes in a variety of textures, the choice of paper will affect the final quality and color of the image. For this reason, it is best to keep the type of photographic paper used consistent in images produced for longitudinal studies.

Photographic films are produced from negatives. Negative strips are numbered and can be easily stored and filed with appropriate patient codes and information for easy long-term retrieval.

Photographic prints can also be scanned and stored as digital images by means of a computer scanner. High-quality scanned photographic prints are often equal to or of higher visual quality than images produced by digital cameras. Photographic prints can be viewed without special equipment, and copies can be stored directly in the patient's case folder for easy review. Photographic prints can also be reproduced as 35 mm slides.

Digital Images

As previously mentioned, slide transparencies and photographs can be digitally stored and viewed on computer monitors. Digital photography is becoming more popular in medical centers because of its convenience, storage capacity, ease of operation, and ability to be transferred to and viewed on a computer. Initial concerns about clinical quality of digital photographs are becoming less of an issue as digital technology improves. Recent studies comparing image quality have suggested that digital imaging of high-quality digital cameras is equal to, and for some purposes, better than traditional images produced by SLR photography (Barker, et al., 1998; Becker, Svensson, & Jacobsson, 1998). Because digital cameras record and store digital images directly on floppy computer disks without the need for film, they are a good choice when archival storage of large numbers of photographs is needed. The drawback is that digital images are most effectively viewed on a computer with a large memory capacity, and a high-resolution monitor. Digital images can be printed out, but the printed images must be protected from direct sunlight and moisture. Quality of the printed images varies with the quality of the printer and the printer paper.

Lighting Conditions

Lighting is among the least controllable of photographic conditions. All photographers have experienced the frustration of preparing to photograph a special event only to have those plans altered by the absence of sufficient light or the presence of too much light for optimal photographic conditions. The subject of selecting and preparing photographic lighting is too extensive to be addressed thoroughly in this text. For most SLPs, the most effective, versatile, and affordable lighting choice is electronic flash. This subject is discussed in detail below.

Electronic Flash

Most types of film are called "daylight" film, because they are designed to respond to sunlight, or to the light from an electronic flash that duplicates the conditions of sunlight. When daylight film is used indoors without electronic flash the resulting photograph may have an unusual color cast to it. For example, photographs taken indoors under fluorescent lights will appear to be greenish. Professional photographers correct such problems by using special indoor films, light meters, studio lighting, and color correction filters.

Photographers who have neither the time nor the funds to invest in professional lighting systems and who do not wish to purchase or use special films or filters must rely on electronic flash systems. Modern through the lens (TTL) flash units are designed for use with SLR cameras. Because these flash units "read" information coming in from the camera, the correct lighting is automatically adjusted for each photographic situation.

Electronic flash systems are a good choice for medical photography because they provide balanced, consistent lighting and are generally easy to operate. Flash attachments are usually mounted on top of the camera—a convenient location, but not always the most photographically desirable one. Some flash attachments allow the user to manipulate the flash head and "bounce" the light off a reflective surface. "Bounced" lighting is often less harsh than light projected directly onto the subject from a top-mounted flash.

More experienced photographers may prefer to mount two flash units on a bracket and connect them to the camera with cords. Figure 7–2 shows such a flash system. The camera is placed in the center of the bracket. The flash units can be placed in almost any position relative to the subject. Side-mounted flash units are especially effective in photographing eyes. The curvature and depth of eyes may be lost when photographing with a macro lens using top-mounted flash. Dual flash units mounted on brackets maintain depth of field and give accurate color rendition in such cases. Because both flash units are reflected by the eye, the resulting photograph gives the subject's eyes an unnatural appearance for portrait photography.

Flash units and cameras are battery powered. When a flash is operated extensively, batteries can be depleted quickly. Always have spare flash and camera batteries on hand, especially when large numbers of photographs are planned.

In summary, SLPs who plan to use photography for educational or diagnostic purposes should select equipment according to their specific needs and employment situation. Special cameras, lenses, film, and lighting exist for almost every budget and photographic situation. Once appropriate equipment is available, photographic protocols should be established and maintained.

TAKING ACCURATE PATIENT PHOTOGRAPHS

Professional photographers are accustomed to hearing the phrase, "What a great photograph! You must have a really good camera." Persons making this good-intentioned, but erroneous remark assume that high-quality equipment guarantees photographic success. Although equipment is a factor, successful clinical photography also depends on the photographer's purpose, organizational skills, photographic experience, and ethical behavior.

Photographic Purpose

Health care professionals should have a clear purpose for photographing patients. Photographing for the sake of photographing uses time that could be better spent in direct diagnostic or therapy procedures. Nonetheless, when specific diagnostic, educational, or research needs have been identified, health care professionals are justified in using photography to meet those needs. Before photographing any patient ask yourself the following questions: Why am I taking this photograph? Will this photograph accomplish my purpose? Is it in the patient's best interest

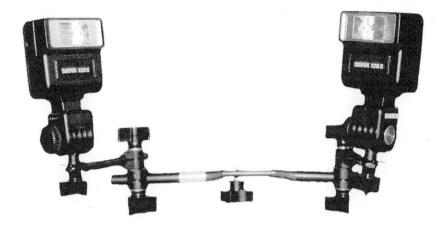

Figure 7–2. A bracket flash system.

to be photographed? How will this photograph be used? Unless photography clearly contributes to better patient safety, diagnosis, or treatment, then time spent in this activity is probably not justified.

Using time expeditiously is necessary, even when photography *is* justified. Photographic sessions can be shortened by using good organizational skills and by becoming familiar with equipment through extensive practice.

Organizational Skills

Table 7–2 summarizes general and specific tips for photographing patients. The most important of these is to have a specific photographic protocol and to follow it consistently. Implementing a consistent plan is considerably easier if materials and equipment are organized and operational well before the photographic session begins. This is easier to accomplish when photography is done in a consistent location. Although a formal photographic studio is desirable, it is not necessary for the production of high-quality photographs. It is possible to create good photographic conditions by selecting a well-lit area with a nonreflective background. Background cloth such as imitation suede is easy to transport and can function as a backdrop, even in congested surroundings. Before beginning, be sure that the equipment is working and that spare film and batteries are easily accessible. Although through the lens flash systems guarantee consistent lighting conditions, select the brightest lit location to prevent "red eye." Red eye is more likely to occur when the subject's pupils are widely dilated. Photographing in well-lit areas causes

Table 7–2. Tips for Photographing Patients

General Photographic Issues

- Have a consistent photography protocol. Select appropriate equipment and use it in subsequent photography sessions as long as it is available and in good working order.

- Have a photography area organized and ready before the patient arrives. Keep spare film, batteries, and equipment on hand in case of equipment failure.

- Work systematically and quickly. Be considerate of patients who are sick, developmentally delayed, or who have attention deficit disorders. Discontinue photography session if patient shows signs of psychological distress.

- Remember that babies and young children may be frightened by flash attachments and that electronic flash is sometimes uncomfortable for older persons and persons with cataracts.

- Keep detailed written records. Data sheets listing patient code names, film type, body parts photographed, lighting conditions, and date of photography should be maintained and filed.

- Make back-up copies of written records and photographs and store these on computer disks.

- Keep negatives in archival plastic sleeves and store prints in acid-free containers.

- Store back-up computer disks, negatives, and prints in a dust-free, heat-and-humidity controlled environment.

Specific Photographic Techniques

- If photos are to be used in longitudinal studies, request that patients remove makeup and jewelry before coming to photo session. Inform patients that their hair may be moved aside to photograph hairline, neckline, or ear placement.

- Photograph each patient from front, posterior, superior views, and both profiles.

- Photograph full body from same distance each session. Use tape marks on floor to control distance between photographer and subject.

- Photograph individual features (eyes, ears, nose) at the same level as the feature. Keep the film plane parallel to the feature you are photographing.

- Turning off the autofocus feature often makes focusing on eyes and ears easier.

- Keep the level of ambient lighting as high as possible to avoid red eye.

- Photograph consistently; for example, if patients were originally photographed without makeup, continue that practice in future photographs.

- Use a smooth, nonreflective backdrop. If a backdrop is unavailable, position patient in front of a nontextured, nonreflective, neutrally colored surface.

- End the photo session by taking one portrait, an informal photograph for the patient's enjoyment.

the subject's pupils to constrict, reducing the chance of recording a red reflection from the subject's retina.

Photographic Experience

Familiarity with equipment operation will also expedite the photography session. Photographic innovations such as autofocus can simplify photography, but use of such special features also requires practice to implement successfully. For example, in some instances, manual focus will achieve the desired result more effectively than autofocus. Only through practice can the photographer learn to select the best photographic options. Operating an SLR camera quickly and accurately takes considerable practice. Although basic familiarity with equipment will probably be sufficient to produce acceptable photographs, even experienced photographers may wish to learn advanced photographic techniques for close-up patient photography. Current articles on patient photography are often found in dental and surgical journals. Articles by DiBernardo, Adams, Krause, Fiorillo, and Gheradini (1998) and Dorfman (1995) provide a good starting point in learning advanced photographic techniques.

Photographic Ethics

All photographs to be used for clinical, research, or educational purposes require written permission from the patient or the patient's caregiver. Separate photographic consent forms should be used for children, for adults, and for adults who require a caregiver's consent. Table 7–3 illustrates a generic permission form for photographing children. Although a form's content and style may vary depending on a given work setting's policies, all such forms should contain:

- basic identifying information
- the purpose of the photographic session
- a statement of how resulting images are to be used
- a statement of patient's privacy rights
- an indication of specific body parts to be photographed
- assurances that the subject may withdraw consent without penalty at any time

Consent forms should be reviewed with the photographic subject and or his or her family members, dated, signed by the photographer

Table 7–3. Example of Written Authorization to Photograph Patient

National University Speech and Hearing Clinic

100 Forest Avenue

Biggsville, Ohio

Photographic Consent Form for Children

I _____ (parent or guardian) consent that photographic and/or video pictures may be taken of my child under the following conditions:

The photographs and/or video pictures shall be used for clinical records. If, in the judgment of _____ (name of investigator), medical research, education, or science will be benefited by their use, such pictures and information relating to my child may be published and republished either separately or in connection with each other, in professional journals, medical books, or textbooks, or may be transmitted by television, computer Internet, or other device for viewing. They may also be used for any other purpose which _____ (name of investigator) may deem proper in the interest of medical education, knowledge, or research; provided, however, that it is specifically understood that in any such publication or use, my child shall not be identified by name.

The aforementioned photographs and/or video pictures may be modified or retouched in any way that the researcher, in his or her discretion, may consider desirable. I _____ (parent or guardian) have been given a complete description of the procedures to be used in this photographic session, and I agree that my child may participate in the procedures.

I understand the use for the medical photographs in areas of education, research, and patient care, and I give permission to _____ (name of investigator) to use the photographs at his or her discretion.

I am aware that all measures to protect my child's privacy and anonymity will be maintained.

I am aware that I may withdraw my consent at any time during the photographic procedure without prejudice or penalty of jeopardizing the care my child receives.

I give permission for photographs to be taken of (initial all which apply) my child's ___ eyes ___ ears ___ head ___ neck ___ face ___ hands ___ feet ___ other_____ (specified).

I have read and understand my child's rights and obligations as stated in the above consent form. I thereby give my permission to _____ (name of investigator) to obtain photographs of _____ (name of child) and use them according to his or her discretion. I realize that I may withdraw my child at any time without jeopardizing the care he or she receives in any way.

Name of Subject	Date	Witness	Date

Name of Parent or Guardian _____

and the subject or the subject's caregiver, and witnessed by someone who is unrelated to the photographer and the photographic subject. The patients or caregiver should receive a copy of the consent form, and the original should be kept in the photographer's records.

Technically, photographers may publish photographs if the human subject cannot be identified (a photograph of an eye, for example). Nonetheless, it is good practice to obtain written permission for all photographs taken for educational purposes. In the past, photographers sometimes blacked out portions of photographs to assure patient anonymity. This practice is no longer recommended, and in any case it produces distracting photographic images.

Photographic consent forms serve as a legal contract between photographer and subject. Even after a patient gives photographic consent, there is considerable photographic flexibility within the terms of most consent forms. This flexibility raises ethical questions about photographic honesty and patient safety (Table 7–4).

Photographic Honesty

Photographers have always had the ability to enhance, manipulate, and change the appearance of photographic images by use of lighting, filters, and darkroom techniques. Portrait photographers, whose goal is to make the subject look as attractive as possible, make liberal use of such techniques to create pleasing photographic images. Clinical photographers, on the other hand, seek *accuracy* of photographic images, especially when those images will be used for accessing results of dental or surgical procedures. Health care professionals should be extremely careful to present results as honestly as possible, and to evaluate photographs in medical literature in terms of honesty of presentation. Consider for example, pre- and postoperative photographs of a teenager who has a facial anomaly appearing side by side in a surgical journal. The first, preoperative photograph shows an unsmiling woman wearing a white hospital smock. She wears no makeup or jewelry, and her hair is pulled back from her face, clearly revealing her ears and facial anomaly. The adjacent photograph taken one year following surgical correction of the facial anomaly shows a smiling woman with an attractive hairstyle that covers her ears and obscures most of her cheeks. She is wearing colorful clothing that enhance her skin tone and makeup that covers her surgical scars. Although both photographs were taken under identical conditions using identical equipment, film and lighting, do they *accurately* reflect the effectiveness of surgical remediation for the facial anomaly? Is such a comparison an *illegal* use of photography? Is this an *ethical* way to report surgical results?

Table 7–4. Ethical Considerations

Relationships with Patients

- Always ask permission before photographing anyone.
- Obtain signed, witnessed written photographic permission before photographing.
- Be considerate of the patient's feelings. Remember you are photographing an person, not an anomaly or a body part.
- Prepare to spend time explaining purpose and procedures of the photographic session.
- Be certain the patient or caregiver understands that he or she may withdraw consent for use of patient photographs at any time without penalty.

Patient Safety

- Ask patient to remove or conceal identifiable information such as name tags, monograms, or initialed jewelry.
- Leave photography of sensitive issues (child abuse, birth anomalies involving genitals) to professional medical photographers.
- Make patient safety a priority. Be cautious about placing patient photographs on the Internet.
- Use code numbers or pseudonyms when referring to photographs of patients during lectures or in publications.
- If photographs of patients are used to illustrate lectures, be sure they serve a specific purpose and are treated respectfully in discussions with the audience.

Photography Honesty

- If photographs are significantly altered from original appearance, clearly state the nature of these changes in publications or in discussions with a viewing audience.
- Make every effort to maintain consistent photographic conditions when recording longitudinal changes in the patient's appearance.
- Resist the temptation to digitally alter the final appearance of photographs. Remember that the goal of scientific photography is to accurately record the patient's appearance, not attractively record the patient's appearance.

Such pre- and postoperative photography is still common practice, and, in justice to the majority of health care professionals, is probably not deliberately intended to deceive. Today, however, digital imaging software has made it possible for anyone with a computer and the appropriate software to retouch, enhance, resize or crop photographic images on screen. Sophisticated, costly digital imaging programs such as Adobe Photoshop also allow the user to distort, change, or "paste" one photographic image onto another.

From a positive point of view, digital imaging programs provide a way to improve photographic quality without compromising the integrity of the original image. Many of the photographs in this text, for example, have been digitally altered to remove background material. This was done to eliminate distracting material that contributed nothing to the appearance of the subject.

The negative side of such technology is that digital imaging programs make it possible to create craniofacial anomalies where none exist; to "erase" craniofacial anomalies where they do exist; to change the color of eyes, skin, and hair; and in short, to deliberately alter photographic images for unethical and, in some cases, illegal purposes.

To prevent photographic misinterpretation of digitally altered photographs, the photographer should state if and how photographic images have been changed from the original. Having permission to take clinical photographs is not a license to deliberately alter photographic outcomes. Where photographic enhancement stops and photographic deception begins depends largely on the judgment and ethical standards of the individual photographer.

Patient Safety

Health care professionals have an obligation to see that photographic materials are used only in accordance with the purposes agreed upon in the photographic release, and to insure that such use does not compromise the safety of the patients who have agreed to be photographed.

A quick tour of the Internet reveals hundreds of Web sites created by parents or family members of individuals who have craniofacial anomalies and genetic syndromes. Many Web sites are illustrated by photographs of affected individuals and their families. Those families obviously wish to share information with similarly affected families, as well as to educate the public in general about specific disorders and their ramifications.

Health care professionals may be lulled into the belief that because such practices are common, they are safe, educational, and worthy of imitation. Placing a patient's photograph in a textbook differs from placing a patient's photograph on a Web site, even if both the textbook and the Web site exist for sound educational purposes.

Web sites can theoretically be accessed by anyone in the world. Information on those Web sites can be copied, cut and pasted, digitally altered, and transmitted over E-mail almost instantaneously. Photographs from Web sites can be converted into screen savers or backgrounds for computer screens, letterheads, photographs for brochures, logos for athletic equipment—the list of possibilities is endless. Is it *ethical* to place a patient's photograph on a Web site, even if we have written permission to do so? Is it *safe* to put that person's photograph in a place that can be accessed by anyone, regardless of educational background, intelligence, or criminal background? Digital photographs on the Internet have the capacity to educate, inform, and allow individuals with craniofacial anomalies to interact with persons who share similar problems. What is the appropriate boundary between patient safety and patient education? These questions, and others like them, have not been satisfactorily addressed by the health care professions, and no wide spread agreement on what constitutes "computer safety" has yet been accepted. Until there are specific guidelines, it is probably best to employ a conservative approach to publication of patient photographs on the Internet.

SUMMARY

Photography is a valuable skill that allows health care professionals to visually diagnose craniofacial anomalies, to keep visual records for patient safety, to observe longitudinal changes, and to prepare educational materials. A variety of camera types are available to suit any photographic purpose. Through the careful selection of camera, film, lighting, and accessory equipment a basic photography protocol can be developed for systematic photography of patients in almost any employment setting.

Health care professionals should have a clear purpose for photographing patients, be organized, and ideally have experience photographing a variety of situations. All photography depicting recognizable human subjects requires subject consent. Patients must provide written consent before photography begins and must be given the opportunity to withdraw such consent at any time without penalty. Written consent does not excuse photographers from behaving ethically. Persons who take medical photographs are ethically, if not legally, responsible for the safety and well being of the individuals they photograph.

REFERENCES

Barker, N. J., Zahurak, M., Olson, J. L., Nadasdy, T., Racusen, L. C., & Hruban, R. H. (1998). Digital imaging of black-and-white photomicrographs: impact of file size. *American Journal of Surgical Pathology, 22* ,1411–1416.

Becker, M., Svensson, H., & Jacobsson, S. (1998). Clinical examination compared with morphometry of digital photographs for evaluation of repaired cleft lips. *Scandinavian Journal of Plastic and Reconstructive Surgery and Hand Surgery, 32*, 301–306.

DiBernardo, B. E., Adams, R. L., Krause, J., Fiorillo, M. A., & Gheradini, G. (1998). Photographic standards in plastic surgery. *Plastic and Reconstructive Surgery, 102,* 559–568.

Dorfman, W. M. (1995). Inexpensive high-quality full-face patient photographs. *Dentistry Today, 14,* 54.

Fann, P. P. (1998a). Choosing the right clinical camera. Part I. *Oral Health, 88*(4), 67–69, 71, 73.

Fann, P. P. (1998b). Choosing the right clinical camera. Part II. *Oral Health, 88*(5), 35–39, 41–42.

Fann, P. P. (1998c). Choosing the right clinical camera. Part III. *Oral Health, 88*(6), 35–39, 41–42.

APPENDIX

SYNDROMES WITH COMMUNICATION DISORDERS

Syndromes With Communication Disorders	Speech	Resonance	Voice	Language	Hearing Sensorineural	Conductive
Aarskog-Scott Syndrome additional features include hypodontia, brachydactyly, short stature, small nose, broad philtrum, crease below the lower lip, maxillary hypoplasia, broad central upper incisors, cognitive impairment, ADD, ptosis of eyelids, downslanting palpebral fissures, widow's peak, hypertelorism	•	•		•		
Aicardi's Syndrome additional features include microphthalmia, brain anomalies, cleft lip, cleft palate, microcephaly, partial to total agenesis of corpus collosum, cognitive impairment, optic nerve coloboma, spina bifida, rib anomalies, iris coloboma	•	•		•		
Albright's Hereditary Osteodystrophy Syndrome additional features include cognitive impairment, cataracts, rounded face, brachydactyly, obesity, small stature, low nasal bridge, delayed dental eruption, enamel hypoplasia, anomalous digits, prognathic profile, vertebral defects, hearing deficit, short limbs, large great toe, small, upturned nose, hypoplastic maxilla, short neck	•	•		•		•
Angelman's Syndrome additional features include microcephaly, ataxic arm movements, seizures, cognitive impairment, decreased pigmentation of iris and choroid, maxillary hypoplasia, widely spaced teeth, blond hair, pale blue eyes, optic atrophy, macrostomia, prognathic mandible, inappropriate laughter, absent speech, large fontanels, macrostomia	•					
Antley-Bixler Syndrome additional features include digital anomalies, kidney anomalies, heart anomalies, proptosis, frontal bossing, dysplastic ears, depressed nasal bridge, craniosynostosis, brachycephaly, large anterior fontanel, radio-humeral synostosis, femoral bowing, midface hypoplasia, stenotic external auditory canals, finger and joint anomalies, delayed closure of fontanels	•	•		•		•

	Speech	Resonance	Voice	Language	Hearing Sensorineural	Hearing Conductive
Apert's Syndrome additional features include syndactyly, hydrocephalus, cognitive impairment, hypertelorism, high forehead, large fontanels with late closure, strabismus, small nose, narrow palate with median groove, downslanting palpebral fissures, occasional cleft palate, irregular craniosynostosis, fusion of cervical vertebrae, flat facies, shallow orbits, nystagmus, short anterio-posterior craniofacial diameter	•	•	•	•		•
Basal-Cell Nevus Syndrome additional features include macrocephaly, scoliosis, strabismus, basal cell carcinomas, frontoparietal bossing, broad nasal bridge, prognathism, occasional cognitive impairment, sloping narrow shoulders, vertebral anomalies, heavy fused eyebrows, misshapen carious teeth, epidermal cysts, nevi, nystagmus	•	•		•		
Beckwith-Wiedemann Syndrome additional features include large size at birth, hypotonia, accelerated growth, macroglossia, creases in ear lobes, large ears, preauricular tags and pits, enlarged liver, enlarged spleen, enlarged kidneys, prominent eyes, large fontanels, malocclusion, prognathic mandible, macrosomia, capillary nevus flammeus	•	•	•	•		•
Berardinelli-Lipodystrophy Syndrome additional features include enlarged liver and heart, cognitive impairment, hirsutism, muscular hypertrophy, tall stature, coarse skin, large superficial veins, absence of facial subcutaneous fat, hypertrophic tonsils and adenoids, curly scalp hair, accelerated growth and maturation, enlarged hands and feet, hyperpigmentation	•	•		•		
Bixler's Syndrome additional features include hypertelorism, short stature, cleft lip, cleft palate, heart anomalies, frontal bossing, craniosynostosis, microtia, depressed nasal bridge, dysplastic ears, anomalous ossicles, cognitive impairment	•	•		•		•

	Speech	Resonance	Voice	Language	Hearing Sensorineural	Conductive
Blepharonasofacial Syndrome additional features include telecanthus, broad nasal root, cognitive impairment, midface hypoplasia, hyperextensible joints, cup-shaped ears, hypertelorism	•			•		
Bloch-Sulzberger Syndrome/ Incontinentia Pigmenti Syndrome additional features include strabismus, hypodontia, central nervous system anomalies, alopecia, retinal detachment, cataracts, microcephaly, mental deficiency, nystagmus, coarse hair, sparse hair in early childhood, linear distribution of blisters along limbs and trunk, hyperpigmentation on lines of Blaschko	•			•		
Bloom's Syndrome additional features include short stature, cognitive deficiency, psychiatric illness, deficient subcutaneous fat, microcephaly, molar hypoplasia, facial erythema, hypopigmentation, hyperpigmentation, café au lait spots	•		•	•		
Cardio-Facio-Cutaneous Syndrome additional features include large forehead, sparse curly scalp hair, depressed nasal root, short neck, ptosis, small stature, hypotonia, cardiac anomalies, posteriorly rotated ears, nystagmus, strabismus, mild-to-moderate mental retardation, shallow orbital ridges, brain anomalies, relative macrocephaly, downslanting palpebral fissures	•	•	•	•		
Carpenter's Syndrome additional features include hypertelorism, polydactyly, cognitive impairment, heart anomalies, lateral displacement of inner canthi, inner canthal folds, craniosynostosis, small stature, flat nasal bridge, optic atrophy, obesity, variable synostosis, brachydactyly of hands, low set malformed ears, high arched palate, large fontanels	•	•		•		

	Speech	Resonance	Voice	Language	Hearing Sensorineural	Conductive
Cat Eye Syndrome additional features include iris coloboma, hypertelorism, cognitive impairment, short stature, anal anomalies, hernias, downslanting palpebral fissures, micrognathia, preauricular pits and tags, cardiac defects	•	•		•		•
CHARGE Syndrome additional features include iris coloboma, heart anomalies, choanal atresia, growth retardation, ear anomalies, genital anomalies, nystagmus, micrognathia, cleft lip, facial palsy, mental deficiency, short neck	•	•	•	•	•	•
Clouston's Syndrome additional features include thickened skin on palms and feet, strabismus, short stature, alopecia, hypoplastic nails, hyperpigmentation, deficient eyelashes and eyebrows	•			•		
Cockayne's Syndrome additional features include microcephaly, progressive cognitive impairment, central hearing impairment, optic atrophy, retinal pigmentation anomalies, hypotelorism, nystagmus, profound postnatal growth deficiency, dental abnormalities, ataxia, dysarthic speech, seizures, loss of adipose tissue	•	•	•	•	•	
Coffin-Lowry/Coffin-Siris Syndrome additional features include coarse facies, small stature, hypotonia, puffy hands, hypodontia, full lips, downslanting palpebral fissures, maxillary hypoplasia, short broad nose, prominent ears, growth deficiency, macrostomia, tapering fingers, coarse appearance, hypertelorism	•			•		
Cohens's Syndrome additional features include short stature, cognitive impairment, hypotonia, obesity, scoliosis, narrow face, downslanting palpebral fissures, high nasal root, downslanting eyes, microcephaly, decreased visual acuity, narrow hands and feet, simian creases, hyperextensible joints, delayed puberty, prominent maxillary incisors, high narrow palate, large ears	•			•		

	Speech	Resonance	Voice	Language	Hearing Sensorineural	Hearing Conductive
Crouzon's Syndrome additional features include macrocephaly, maxillary hypoplasia, hypertelorism, frontal bossing, upslanting palpebral fissures, low set ears, hypoplastic maxilla, ocular proptosis, nystagmus, mental retardation, iris coloboma, strabismus, optic atrophy, inverted V shape to palate, craniosynostosis	•	•				•
DeBarsy's Syndrome additional features include small stature, cognitive impairment, wrinkled skin, athetosis, hypotonia, microcephaly, large ears	•			•		
DeLange's Syndrome additional features include short stature, limb reduction, depressed nasal bridge, microcephaly, hypertonia, cleft palate, low anterior hairline, thin upper lip, short neck, micrognathia, long curly eyelashes, downturned corners of mouth, high arched palate, mental retardation, bushy eyebrows, hirsutism, clinodactyly of fifth fingers, simian creases, blue sclera, nystagmus, downslanting palpebral fissures	•	•	•	•	•	•
Ellis-van Creveld Syndrome additional features include short stature, short limbs, anodontia, short upper lip, labial frenula, dysplastic nails, cleft palate, prominent nose, narrow palpebral fissures, abundant scalp hair, retruded mandible, neonatal teeth, short upper lip, polydactyly of fingers, short broad middle phalanges, iris coloboma	•			•		
Fanconi's Pancytopenia Syndrome additional features include short stature, microcephaly, small or absent thumbs, renal anomalies, strabismus, hypoplastic radii, cognitive impairment, eye anomalies, nystagmus, hyperpigmentation	•			•		•
Femoral-Facial Syndrome additional features include cleft palate, micrognathia, upslanting palpebral fissures, short nose, thin upper lip, ear anomalies	•	•				•

	Speech	Resonance	Voice	Language	Hearing Sensorineural	Conductive
Fetal Alcohol Syndrome additional features include growth deficiency, low birth weight, microcephaly, short palpebral fissures, short nose, cleft palate, maxillary hypoplasia, smooth philtrum with thin and smooth upper lip, cognitive impairment, joint anomalies, hypertelorism, protruding ears, numerous hair whorls	•	•	•	•		•
Fetal Hydantoin Syndrome additional features include growth deficiency, cleft palate, cleft lip, short nose, flat philtrum, low anterior hairline, hypoplastic distal phalanges, hirsutism, wide anterior fontanel, ocular hypertelorism, broad nasal bridge, bowed upper lip, cognitive impairment, short neck, abnormal palmar crease, coarse hair, low posterior hairline, upslanting palpebral fissures, delayed closure of fontanels	•	•		•		•
Fraser's Syndrome additional features include syndactyly, small and abnormal genitals, scalp hair on forehead, cognitive impairment, cryptophthalmos, broad nose with depressed bridge, hypoplastic nares, hypertelorism, cup-shaped ears	•		•	•		
Freeman-Sheldon Syndrome additional features include mask-like face, micrognathia, ulnar deviation of fingers, limited oral opening, broad nasal bridge, telecanthus, strabismus, small nose, small tongue, epicanthal folds, small mouth, deep set eyes, joint anomalies, downslanting palpebral fissures, hypertelorism	•	•				•
Frontonasal Dysplasia Sequence additional features include hypertelorism, cleft lip, strabismus, prominent forehead, broad nasal bridge, small mandible, flexion defects of fingers, coarse facies, partial anodontia, widow's peak, hypotelorism	•	•		•	•	•

	Speech	Resonance	Voice	Language	Hearing Sensorineural	Conductive
Goltz's Syndrome additional features include skin and nail anomalies, strabismus, small eyes, nystagmus, small stature, cognitive impairment, hypoplastic teeth, microphthalmus, syndactyly of fingers and/or toes, narrow nasal bridge, ear anomalies, sparse brittle hair, iris coloboma, asymmetric hands and feet	•			•		
Hallermann-Streiff Syndrome additional features include short stature, micrognathia, small face, thin small pointed nose, nystagmus, sparse scalp hair and eyelashes, frontal and parietal bossing, cataracts, hypoplastic teeth, microphthalmia, blue sclera, alopecia, hypotelorism, iris coloboma, microstomia, downslanting palpebral fissures, delayed closure of fontanels	•	•	•			
Holoprosencephaly additional features include absent bipolar development of brain, absence of olfactory bulbs and tracts, microcephaly, anosmia, cleft lip or cleft palate, single central incisor, hypotelorism	•	•		•		•
Hurler's Syndrome additional features include short stature, dementia, coarse facial features, short neck, macroencephaly, corneal clouding, full lips, flared nostrils, low nasal bridge, inner epicanthal folds, retinal pigmentation, cognitive impairment, large tongue, small teeth, joint anomalies, heart anomalies, hirsutism, nystagmus, iris coloboma	•	•	•	•	•	
Hypohidrotic Ectodermal Dysplasia Syndrome additional features include thin fair skin, hypopigmentation, alopecia, sparse fine hair, silver hair, hypodontia, small nose, thin and wrinkled eyelids, hypoplastic sweat glands, conical anterior teeth, full forehead, low nasal bridge, full lips	•		•			

	Speech	Resonance	Voice	Language	Hearing Sensorineural	Conductive
Kabuki Make-Up Syndrome additional features include cognitive impairment, long palpebral fissures, large protruding ears, short stature, cleft lip, cleft palate, arching eyebrows, finger anomalies, postnatal growth deficiency, preauricular pits and tags, tooth anomalies, open mouth	•	•	•	•		•
Klinefelter's Syndrome additional features include micropenis, cleft palate, obesity, elbow dysplasia, fifth finger clinodactyly, long limbs, tall slim stature, behavior problems, iris coloboma, upslanting palpebral fissures	•			•		
LEOPARD Syndrome additional features include hypertelorism, multiple lentigines, electrocardiographic conduct abnormalities, pulmonic stenosis, abnormal genitalia, mild growth deficiency, protruding ears, cryptorchidism, nystagmus	•	•		•	•	
Louis-Bar's Syndrome additional features include athetosis, progressive ataxia, progressive cognitive deterioration, nystagmus, small stature, telangiectasia over bridge of nose and auricles, café au lait spots	•	•	•	•		
Lowe's Syndrome additional features include cataracts, nystagmus, hypotonia, cognitive impairment, renal dysfunction, cryptochordism, osteoporosis	•			•		
Marfan's Syndrome additional features include tall stature, abnormal skeletal growth pattern, hyperextensible joints, hypotonia, myopia, retinal detachment, nystagmus, blue sclera, iris coloboma, arachnodactyly, narrow facies with narrow palate, hernias	•	•				
Marinesco-Sjögren Syndrome additional features include microcephaly, small stature, cognitive impairment, ataxia, cataracts, ichthyosis, hypertelorism, nystagmus	•	•		•		

	Speech	Resonance	Voice	Language	Hearing Sensorineural	Hearing Conductive
Möbius Syndrome additional features include small mouth, micrognathia, hypoglossia, cleft palate, broad nose, telecanthus, facial asymmetry, hypodontia, high nasal bridge, downslanting palpebral fissures	•	•		•		
Morquio's Syndrome additional features include short stature, corneal clouding, joint and spine anomalies, short neck, macrostomia, short nose, widely spaced teeth, coarse facial features, thin enamel on teeth, deep central dimple in chin		•	•		•	•
Nager's Syndrome additional features include micrognathia, cleft or absent palate, external and middle-ear anomalies, hair on lateral cheek, downslanting palpebral fissures, absent lower eyelashes, atresia of external ear canal, high nasal bridge, preauricular tags	•	•				•
Neurofibromatosis-Type I additional features include café au lait spots, cutaneous neurofibromas, skeletal anomalies, pigmented iris, heterochromia	•	•	•	•		
Neurofibromatosis-Type II additional features include bilateral acoustic neuromas, CNS tumors, pigmented iris, short stature, cutaneous neurofibromas, heterochromia, café au lait spots	•				•	
Neurofibromatosis-Type III additional features include CNS tumors, acoustic neuromas, macroencephaly, optic glioma, short stature, café au lait spots, heterochromia	•			•	•	
Noonan's Syndrome additional features include short stature, ptosis of eyelids, low posterior hairline, webbed neck, short neck, downslanting eyes, cardiac defect, epicanthal folds, hypertelorism, myopia, nystagmus, strabismus, malocclusion, cognitive impairment, wide mouth, prominent upper lip, retrognathia, low set ears, downslanting palpebral fissures	•	•	•	•	•	•

	Speech	Resonance	Voice	Language	Hearing Sensorineural	Conductive
Oculo-Auriculo-Vertebral Spectrum additional features include facial asymmetry, spine anomalies, hypoplastic facial musculature, middle-ear anomalies, microtia, cleft palate, facial paresis, macrostomia, preauricular tags and pits, tongue anomalies, deep central dimple in chin, hypotelorism, iris coloboma, downslanting palpebral fissures	•	•	•	•		•
Oculo-Dento-Digital Syndrome additional features include microphthalmia, hypotelorism, small corneas, short palpebral fissures, epicanthal folds, small nares, sparse hair with abnormal texture, broad lower jaw, alopecia, enamel hypoplasia, syndactyly of fourth and fifth fingers	•				•	
Opitz's Syndrome additional features include cleft palate, cleft lip, upward or downward slanting palpebral fissures, ocular hypertelorism, broad nasal bridge, short neck, cryptorchidism, hypospadias, widow's peak, posterior rotation of auricle, mild-to-moderate mental retardation, hypotelorism	•	•	•	•		•
Osteogenesis Imperfecta Type I additional features include bone fragility, blue sclera, small face, small stature, late eruption and irregularly placed teeth, thin skin, otosclerosis, blue gray coloration of teeth, postnatal growth deficiency, triangular facial appearance, delayed closure of fontanels			•		•	•
Oto-Palato-Digital Syndrome, Type I additional features include hypertelorism, downslanting eyes, small stature, cleft soft palate, micrognathia, microstomia, frontal prominence, large fontanels with delayed closure, low set ears, steep naso-basal angulation, small nose, cognitive impairment, hypoplastic facial bones, broad distal phalanges, downslanting palpebral fissures, upslanting palpebral fissures	•	•	•	•		•

	Speech	Resonance	Voice	Language	Hearing Sensorineural	Conductive
Piebaldness additional features include white forelock of hair, hyperpigmented borders between pigmented and unpigmented zones, hypopigmentation	•	•			•	
Prader-Willi Syndrome additional features include short stature, obesity, hypogonadism, hypotonia, small hands and feet, strabismus, blond hair, numerous hair whorls, blue eyes, fair skin, mental retardation, thin upper lip, excessive appetite, almond-shaped palpebral fissures, upslanting palpebral fissures	•	•	•	•		
Proteus Syndrome additional features include enlarged hands and feet, bony projections on skull, large head, multiple hematomas, hyperpigmentation, thickened skin, increased stature, long neck, nevi, unilateral or bilateral overgrowth	•	•		•		•
Pyknodysostosis additional features include short stature, micrognathia, abnormal teeth, osteosclerosis, delayed closure of sutures, delayed closure of fontanels, large fontanels, prominent nose, narrow grooved palate, delayed eruption of teeth			•	•		
Rieger's Syndrome additional features include hypodontia, maxillary deficiency, hernias, broad nasal bridge, thin upper lip, everted lower lip, glaucoma, optic atrophy, iris anomalies, iris coloboma	•					
Robinow's Syndrome additional features include hypertelorism, macrocephaly, cleft palate, brachydactyly, vertebral and skeletal anomalies, short forearms, short stature, prominent eyes, small upturned nose, large anterior fontanel, long philtrum, downslanting palpebral fissures, triangular mouth with downturned angles, micrognathia, crowded teeth, posteriorly rotated ears, alopecia, microstomia, delayed closure of fontanels	•	•				•

	Speech	Resonance	Voice	Language	Hearing Sensorineural	Conductive
Rubinstein-Taybi Syndrome additional features include beaked nose with nasal septum, hypertelorism, cognitive impairment, short stature, downslanting palpebral fissures, hypoplastic maxilla, epicanthal folds, frontal hair upsweep, small mouth, deviated nasal septum, low set and malformed auricles, low posterior-anterior hairline, heavy eyebrows, broad great toes, long eyelashes, epicanthal folds, strabismus, hirsutism, iris coloboma	•		•	•		
Russell-Silver Syndrome additional features include small stature, body asymmetry, large cranium with small triangular face, downturned corners of mouth, late closure of anterior fontanel, micrognathia, hyperhidrosis, hypoglycemia, blue sclera, café au lait spots			•			
Saethre-Chotzen Syndrome additional features include acrocephaly, syndactyly of hands and feet, brachycephaly, high forehead, maxillary hypoplasia, deviated nasal septum, hypertelorism, small ears, ptosis of eyelid, craniosynostosis, large fontanels with delayed closure						•
Scheie's Syndrome additional features include liver enlargement, mild facial coarsening, full lips, broad mouth, deep central dimple in chin, macrostomia, corneal clouding, hirsutism, short neck, prognathic mandible, joint limitations			•			•
Seckel Syndrome additional features include severe short stature, microcephaly, nystagmus, cognitive impairment, micrognathia, receding forehead, prominent nose, low set ears, absent ear lobe, downslanting palpebral fissures, simian crease, digital anomalies	•		•	•		

	Speech	Resonance	Voice	Language	Hearing Sensorineural	Conductive
Soto's Syndrome additional features include large size at birth, large stature, large hands and feet, cognitive impairment, hypotonia, macrocephaly, prominent forehead, large ears, hypertelorism, downslanting palpebral fissures, high narrow palate, premature eruption of teeth, sparse hair, thin brittle fingernails	•		•	•		
Stickler Syndrome additional features include flat facies, micrognathia, cleft palate, low set ears, Robin sequence, depressed nasal bridge, epicanthal folds, mandibular hypoplasia, dental anomalies, prominent eyes, short nose, ocular anomalies, hypotonia, myopia, hyperextensible joints, skeletal anomalies	•	•			•	•
Sturge-Weber Syndrome additional features include seizures, cognitive impairment, cutaneous hemangioma, nevi (usually in a trigeminal facial distribution), limb enlargement, malocclusion	•	•	•	•		
Townes' Syndrome additional features include facial asymmetry, commissural cleft, hemifacial microsomia, preauricular tags and pits, ear tags, microtia, auricular anomalies, hand anomalies					•	
Treacher Collins Syndrome additional features include microtia, downslanting palpebral fissures, micrognathia, absent zygomas, cleft palate, flat frontonasal angle, lower lid coloboma, absent lower eyelashes, malformed auricles, low set ears, preauricular tags and pits, projection of scalp hair onto lateral cheek, molar hypoplasia, mandibular hypoplasia, iris coloboma	•	•				•
Tricho-Rhino-Phalangeal Syndrome, Type I additional features include long nose, sparse hair, small carious teeth, thin nails, short stature, prominent and long philtrum, narrow palate, horizontal groove on chin, malocclusion, mild growth deficiency, digital anomalies, large prominent ears	•		•			

	Speech	Resonance	Voice	Language	Hearing Sensorineural	Conductive
Trisomy 21/Down's Syndrome additional features include upslanted palpebral fissures, short stature, hypotonia, mental retardation, strabismus, short neck, macroglossia, midline parital hair whorl, low posterior hairline, late closure of fontanels, small nose, low nasal bridge, inner epicanthal folds, brushfield spots in iris, hypotelorism, hypertelorism, nystagmus, cardiac anomalies, ear anomalies, protruding ears, microtia	•	•	•	•		•
Turner's Syndrome additional features include short stature, webbed neck, failure of puberty to occur, short neck, low posterior hairline, narrow maxilla, inner canthal folds, downslanting palpebral fissures, obesity, anomalous auricles, narrow palate, excessive pigmented nevi, blue sclera, iris coloboma, hypotelorism			•			•
Velo-Cardio-Facial Syndrome/ DiGeorge's Sequence additional features include short stature, microcephaly, cleft palate, long nose, prominent nose, puffy upper eyelids, nystagmus, squared nasal root, protruding ears, absent earlobes, microtia, vertical maxillary excess, long face, narrow palpebral fissures, downslanting palpebral fissures, abundant scalp hair, slender hands and feet, learning disabilities, heart anomalies, mild intellectual impairment	•	•	•	•	•	•
Waardenburg Syndrome, Type I additional features include heterochromia, partial albinism, pigmentary anomalies of hair, white forelock, hypopigmentation, broad and high nasal bridge, broad mandible, full lips, medial flare of eyebrows, short palpebral fissures					•	
Weaver's Syndrome additional features include thin hair, accelerated growth, skeletal anomalies, large fontanels, macrocephaly, macrostomia, ocular hypertelorism, developmental delay, large protruding ears, camptodactyly, foot deformities, epicanthal folds, long philtrum, broad forehead, downslanting palpebral fissures, coarse and low-pitched voice, progressive spasticity, strabismus	•		•	•		

	Speech	Resonance	Voice	Language	Hearing Sensorineural	Hearing Conductive
Werner's Syndrome additional features include short stature, small hands and feet, beaked nose, premature aging, hyperkeratosis, skin ulcerations, alopecia, sparse gray hair, loss of subcutaneous fat, premature loss of teeth, osteoporosis, hypogonadism, cataracts, retinal degeneration, blue sclera, nystagmus	•			•		
Wildervanck's Syndrome additional features include facial asymmetry, eye motility disorder, nystagmus, epibulbar dermoids, short neck, low hairline, preauricular tags and pits	•	•	•	•	•	•
William's Syndrome additional features include short stature, hypercalcemia, macrostomia, hypertension, hyperopia, hypotelorism, short palpebral fissures, cognitive problems, full lips, hoarse voice, depressed nasal bridge, epicanthal folds, mild microcephaly, medial eyebrow flare, blue eyes, stellate pattern to iris, hyperacusis	•			•		
Wolf-Hirschhorn Syndrome Chromosome 4p Syndrome additional features include microcephaly, cranial asymmetry, ear anomalies, ocular hypertelorism, hypotelorism, short philtrum, cleft lip, cleft palate, strabismus, downslanting palpebral fissures, short hooked nose, iris coloboma, ptosis, nystagmus	•		•	•		
4p- additional features include microcephaly, hypertelorism, ptosis, iris coloboma, broad hooked nose, micrognathia, hypotonia, strabismus, epicanthal folds, downturned corners of mouth, short upper lip and philtrum, preauricular tags and pits, absent earlobes, low posterior hairline, profound mental retardation	•	•	•	•		•
4q+ additional features include microcephaly, short stature, posteriorly rotated ears, low set ears, cleft palate, prominent forehead, downturned corners of mouth	•			•		•

	Speech	Resonance	Voice	Language	Hearing Sensorineural	Conductive
5p+ additional features include small stature, microcephaly, low set ears, hypotonia, seizures, cognitive deficiencies	•		•	•		
5p-/Cri-du-Chat Syndrome additional features include small stature, hypotonia, microcephaly, hypertelorism, epicanthal folds, downslanting palpebral fissures, facial asymmetry, strabismus, preauricular tags and pits, posteriorly rotated ears, low set ears, slow growth, cat-like cry, mental deficiency	•	•	•	•		•
5q+ additional features include microcephaly, large ears, hypertelorism, downslanting eyes, strabismus, micrognathia, cognitive deficiency	•			•		
6q+ additional features include microcephaly, short stature, cleft palate, prominent forehead, downturned corners of mouth, low set ears	•	•	•	•		•
7p- additional features include microcephaly, cognitive deficiency, cranial asymmetry, low set ears depressed nasal root	•	•		•		•
8q+ additional features include cognitive deficiency, short nose, hypertelorism, abnormal skull shape, low set ears	•	•		•		
9p- additional features include hypertelorism, cognitive deficiency, microstomia, micrognathia, ear lobe anomalies, craniosynostosis, short neck, upslanting palpebral fissures, prominent eyes, higher arched eyebrows, depressed nasal bridge, long philtrum, long middle phalanges of fingers	•	•		•		•
11q+ Syndrome additional features include cognitive deficiency, small stature, hypertonia, anal anomalies	•		•	•		

	Speech	Resonance	Voice	Language	Hearing Sensorineural	Conductive
13q- additional features include microcephaly, severe cognitive deficiency, short neck, webbed neck, broad nasal root, frontal bossing, hypertelorism, ptosis, colobomata, epicanthal folds, large slanting ears, microphthalmia	•		•	•		
14q- additional features include hypotonia, seizures, large low set ears, micrognathia	•		•	•		
18p- additional features include small stature, microcephaly, short neck, hypotelorism, retrognathia, deep central dimple in chin, macrostomia, downturned corners of mouth	•	•		•		

Syndromes With Ear Anomalies
Ear Size
Microtia

	Speech	Resonance	Voice	Language	Hearing Sensorineural	Conductive
Bixler's Syndrome additional features include hypertelorism, short stature, cleft lip, cleft palate, heart anomalies, frontal bossing, craniosynostosis, depressed nasal bridge, dysplastic ears, anomalous ossicles, cognitive impairment	•	•		•		•
Oculo-Auriculo-Vertebral Spectrum additional features include facial asymmetry, spine anomalies, hypoplastic facial musculature, middle-ear anomalies, cleft palate, facial paresis, macrostomia, preauricular tags and pits, tongue anomalies, deep central dimple in chin, hypotelorism, iris coloboma, downslanting palpebral fissures	•	•	•	•		•
Towne's Syndrome additional features include facial asymmetry, commissural cleft, hemifacial microsomia, preauricular tags and pits, ear tags, auricular anomalies, hand anomalies					•	
Treacher Collins Syndrome additional features include downslanting palpebral fissures, micrognathia, absent zygomas, cleft palate, flat frontonasal angle, lower lid coloboma, absent lower eyelashes, malformed auricles, low set ears, preauricular tags and pits, projection of scalp hair onto lateral cheek, molar hypoplasia, mandibular hypoplasia, iris coloboma	•	•				•
Trisomy 21/Down's Syndrome additional features include upslanted palpebral fissures, short stature, hypotonia, mental retardation, strabismus, short neck, macroglossia, midline parital hair whorl, low posterior hairline, late closure of fontanels, small nose, low nasal bridge, inner epicanthal folds, brushfield spots in iris, hypotelorism, hypertelorism, nystagmus, cardiac anomalies, ear anomalies, protruding ears	•	•	•	•		•

	Speech	Resonance	Voice	Language	Hearing Sensorineural	Hearing Conductive
Velo-Cardio-Facial Syndrome/ DiGeorge's Sequence additional features include short stature, microcephaly, cleft palate, long nose, prominent nose, puffy upper eyelids, nystagmus, squared nasal root, protruding ears, absent earlobes, vertical maxillary excess, long face, narrow palpebral fissures, downslanting palpebral fissures, abundant scalp hair, slender hands and feet, learning disabilities, heart anomalies, mild intellectual impairment	•	•	•	•	•	•

Large Ears

	Speech	Resonance	Voice	Language	Hearing Sensorineural	Hearing Conductive
Beckwith-Wiedemann Syndrome additional features include large size at birth, hypotonia, accelerated growth, macroglossia, creases in ear lobes, preauricular tags and pits, enlarged liver, enlarged spleen, enlarged kidneys, prominent eyes, large fontanels, malocclusion, prognathic mandible, macrosomia, capillary nevus flammeus	•	•	•	•		•
Coffin-Lowry/Coffin-Siris Syndrome additional features include coarse facies, small stature, hypotonia, puffy hands, hypodontia, full lips, downslanting palpebral fissures, maxillary hypoplasia, short broad nose, growth deficiency, macrostomia, tapering fingers, coarse appearance, hypertelorism	•			•		
Cohen's Syndrome additional features include short stature, cognitive impairment, hypotonia, obesity, scoliosis, narrow face, downslanting palpebral fissures, high nasal root, downslanting eyes, microcephaly, decreased visual acuity, narrow hands and feet, simian creases, hyperextensible joints, delayed puberty, prominent maxillary incisors, high narrow palate	•			•		
DeBarsy's Syndrome additional features include small stature, cognitive impairment, wrinkled skin, athetosis, hypotonia, microcephaly	•			•		

	Speech	Resonance	Voice	Language	Hearing Sensorineural	Conductive
Kabuki Make-Up Syndrome additional features include cognitive impairment, long palpebral fissures, short stature, cleft lip, cleft palate, arching eyebrows, finger anomalies, postnatal growth deficiency, preauricular pits and tags, tooth anomalies, open mouth	•	•	•	•		•
Soto's Syndrome additional features include large size at birth, large stature, large hands and feet, cognitive impairment, hypotonia, macrocephaly, prominent forehead, hypertelorism, downslanting palpebral fissures, high narrow palate, premature eruption of teeth, sparse hair, thin brittle fingernails	•		•	•		
Tricho-Rhino-Phalangeal Syndrome, Type I additional features include long nose, sparse hair, small carious teeth, thin nails, short stature, prominent and long philtrum, narrow palate, horizontal groove on chin, malocclusion, mild growth deficiency, digital anomalies	•		•			
Weaver's Syndrome additional features include thin hair, accelerated growth, skeletal anomalies, large fontanels, macrocephaly, macrostomia, ocular hypertelorism, developmental delay, camptodactyly, foot deformities, epicanthal folds, long philtrum, broad forehead, downslanting palpebral fissures, coarse and low-pitched voice, progressive spasticity, strabismus	•		•	•		
5q+ additional features include microcephaly, hypertelorism, downslanting eyes, strabismus, micrognathia, cognitive deficiency	•			•		
13q- additional features include microcephaly, severe cognitive deficiency, short neck, webbed neck, broad nasal root, frontal bossing, hypertelorism, ptosis, colobomata, epicanthal folds, slanting ears, microphthalmia	•		•	•		
14q- additional features include hypotonia, seizures, low set ears, micrognathia	•		•	•		

Ear Position
Low Set Ears

	Speech	Resonance	Voice	Language	Hearing Sensorineural	Conductive
Crouzon's Syndrome additional features include macrocephaly, maxillary hypoplasia, hypertelorism, frontal bossing, upslanting palpebral fissures, hypoplastic maxilla, ocular proptosis, nystagmus, mental retardation, iris coloboma, strabismus, optic atrophy, inverted V shape to palate, craniosynostosis	•	•				•
Noonan's Syndrome additional features include short stature, ptosis of eyelids, low posterior hairline, webbed neck, short neck, downslanting eyes, cardiac defect, epicanthal folds, hypertelorism, myopia, nystagmus, strabismus, malocclusion, cognitive impairment, wide mouth, prominent upper lip, retrognathia, downslanting palpebral fissures	•	•	•	•	•	•
Oto-Palato-Digital Syndrome, Type I additional features include hypertelorism, downslanting eyes, small stature, cleft soft palate, micrognathia, microstomia, frontal prominence with large fontanels with delayed closure, steep naso-basal angulation, small nose, cognitive impairment, hypoplastic facial bones, broad distal phalanges, downslanting palpebral fissures, upslanting palpebral fissures	•	•	•	•		•
Rubinstein-Taybi Syndrome additional features include beaked nose with nasal septum, hypertelorism, cognitive impairment, short stature, downslanting palpebral fissures, hypoplastic maxilla, epicanthal folds, frontal hair upsweep, small mouth, deviated nasal septum, low set and malformed auricles, low posterior-anterior hairline, heavy eyebrows, broad great toes, long eyelashes, epicanthal folds, strabismus, hirsutism, iris coloboma	•		•	•		
Seckel Syndrome additional features include severe short stature, microcephaly, nystagmus, cognitive impairment, micrognathia, receding forehead, prominent nose, absent ear lobe, downslanting palpebral fissures, simian crease, digital anomalies	•		•	•		

	Speech	Resonance	Voice	Language	Hearing Sensorineural	Conductive
Stickler Syndrome additional features include flat facies, micrognathia, cleft palate, Robin sequence, depressed nasal bridge, epicanthal folds, mandibular hypoplasia, dental anomalies, prominent eyes, short nose, ocular anomalies, hypotonia, myopia, hyperextensible joints, skeletal anomalies	•	•			•	•
Treacher Collins Syndrome additional features include microtia, downslanting palpebral fissures, micrognathia, absent zygomas, cleft palate, flat frontonasal angle, lower lid coloboma, absent lower eyelashes, malformed auricles, preauricular tags and pits, projection of scalp hair onto lateral cheek, molar hypoplasia, mandibular hypoplasia, iris coloboma	•	•				•
5p+ additional features include small stature, microcephaly, hypotonia, seizures, cognitive deficiencies	•		•	•		
5p-/Cri-du-Chat Syndrome additional features include small stature, hypotonia, microcephaly, hypertelorism, epicanthal folds, downslanting palpebral fissures, facial asymmetry, strabismus, preauricular tags and pits, posteriorly rotated ears, slow growth, cat-like cry, mental deficiency	•	•	•	•		•
6q+ additional features include microcephaly, short stature, cleft palate, prominent forehead, downturned corners of mouth	•	•	•	•		•
7p- additional features include microcephaly, cognitive deficiency, cranial asymmetry, depressed nasal root	•	•		•		•
8q+ additional features include cognitive deficiency, short nose, hypertelorism, abnormal skull shape	•	•		•		
14q- additional features include hypotonia, seizures, large ears, micrognathia	•		•	•		

Posteriorly Rotated Ears	Speech	Resonance	Voice	Language	Hearing Sensorineural	Conductive
Cardio-Facio-Cutaneous Syndrome additional features include large forehead, sparse curly scalp hair, depressed nasal root, short neck, ptosis, small stature, hypotonia, cardiac anomalies, nystagmus, strabismus, mild-to-moderate mental retardation, shallow orbital ridges, brain anomalies, relative macrocephaly, downslanting palpebral fissures	•	•	•	•		
Robinow's Syndrome additional features include hypertelorism, macrocephaly, cleft palate, brachydactyly, vertebral and skeletal anomalies, short forearms, short stature, prominent eyes, small upturned nose, large anterior fontanel, long philtrum, downslanting palpebral fissures, triangular mouth with downturned angles, micrognathia, crowded teeth, alopecia, microstomia, delayed closure of fontanels	•	•				•
4q+ additional features include microcephaly, short stature, low set ears, cleft palate, prominent forehead, downturned corners of mouth	•			•		•
5p-/Cri-du-Chat Syndrome additional features include small stature, hypotonia, microcephaly, hypertelorism, epicanthal folds, downslanting palpebral fissures, facial asymmetry, strabismus, preauricular tags and pits, low set ears, slow growth, cat-like cry, mental deficiency	•	•	•	•		•

Ear Orientation
Protruding Ears

	Speech	Resonance	Voice	Language	Hearing Sensorineural	Conductive
Fetal Alcohol Syndrome additional features include growth deficiency, low birth weight, microcephaly, short palpebral fissures, short nose, cleft palate, maxillary hypoplasia, smooth philtrum with thin and smooth upper lip, cognitive impairment, joint anomalies, hypertelorism, numerous hair whorls	•	•	•	•		•

	Speech	Resonance	Voice	Language	Hearing Sensorineural	Hearing Conductive
Kabuki Make-Up Syndrome additional features include cognitive impairment, long palpebral fissures, large ears, short stature, cleft lip, cleft palate, arching eyebrows, finger anomalies, postnatal growth deficiency, preauricular pits and tags, toothanomalies, open mouth	•	•	•	•		•
LEOPARD Syndrome additional features include hypertelorism, multiple lentigines, electrocardiographic conduct abnormalities, pulmonic stenosis, abnormal genitalia, mild growth deficiency, cryptorchidism, nystagmus	•	•		•	•	
Tricho-Rhino-Pharyngeal Syndrome, Type 1 additional features include long nose, sparse hair, small carious teeth, thin nails, short stature, prominent and long philtrum, narrow palate, horizontal groove on chin, malocclusion, mild growth deficiency, digital anomalies, large ears	•		•			
Trisomy 21/Down's Syndrome additional features include upslanted palpebral fissures, short stature, hypotonia, mental retardation, strabismus, short neck, macroglossia, midline parital hair whorl, low posterior hairline, late closure of fontanels, small nose, low nasal bridge, inner epicanthal folds, brushfield spots in iris, hypotelorism, hypertelorism, nystagmus, cardiac anomalies, ear anomalies, microtia	•	•	•	•		•
Velo-Cardio-Facial Syndrome/ DiGeorge's Sequence additional features include short stature, microcephaly, cleft palate, long nose, prominent nose, puffy upper eyelids, nystagmus, squared nasal root, absent earlobes, microtia, vertical maxillary excess, long face, narrow palpebral fissures, downslanting palpebral fissures, abundant scalp hair, slender hands and feet, learning disabilities, heart anomalies, mild intellectual impairment	•	•	•	•	•	•

	Speech	Resonance	Voice	Language	Hearing Sensorineural	Conductive
Weaver's Syndrome additional features include thin hair, accelerated growth, skeletal anomalies, large fontanels, macrocephaly, macrostomia, ocular hypertelorism, developmental delay, large ears, camptodactyly, foot deformities, epicanthal folds, long philtrum, broad forehead, downslanting palpebral fissures, coarse and low-pitched voice, progressive spasticity, strabismus	•		•	•		

Creases in Lobules

	Speech	Resonance	Voice	Language	Hearing Sensorineural	Conductive
Beckwith-Wiedemann Syndrome additional features include large size at birth, hypotonia, accelerated growth, macroglossia, large ears, preauricular tags and pits, enlarged liver, enlarged spleen, enlarged kidneys, prominent eyes, large fontanels, malocclusion, prognathic mandible, macrosomia, capillary nevus flammeus	•	•	•	•		•

Absent Earlobes

	Speech	Resonance	Voice	Language	Hearing Sensorineural	Conductive
Seckel Syndrome additional features include severe short stature, microcephaly, nystagmus, cognitive impairment, micrognathia, receding forehead, prominent nose, low set ears, downslanting palpebral fissures, simian crease, digital anomalies	•		•	•		
Velo-Cardio-Facial Syndrome/ DiGeorge's Sequence additional features include short stature, microcephaly, cleft palate, long nose, prominent nose, puffy upper eyelids, nystagmus, squared nasal root, protruding ears, microtia, vertical maxillary excess, long face, narrow palpebral fissures, downslanting palpebral fissures, abundant scalp hair, slender hands and feet, learning disabilities, heart anomalies, mild intellectual impairment	•	•	•	•	•	•
4p- additional features include microcephaly, hypertelorism, ptosis, iris coloboma, broad hooked nose, micrognathia, hypotonia, strabismus, epicanthal folds, downturned corners of mouth, short upper lip and philtrum, preauricular tags and pits, low posterior hairline, profound mental retardation	•	•	•	•		•

Preauricular Tags and Pits	Speech	Resonance	Voice	Language	Hearing Sensorineural	Conductive
Beckwith-Wiedemann Syndrome additional features include large size at birth, hypotonia, accelerated growth, macroglossia, creases in ear lobes, large ears, enlarged liver, enlarged spleen, enlarged kidneys, prominent eyes, large fontanels, malocclusion, prognathic mandible, macrosomia, capillary nevus flammeus	•	•	•	•		•
Cat Eye Syndrome additional features include iris coloboma, hypertelorism, cognitive impairment, short stature, anal anomalies, hernias, downslanting palpebral fissures, micrognathia, cardiac defects	•	•		•		•
Kabuki Make-Up Syndrome additional features include cognitive impairment, long palpebral fissures, large protruding ears, short stature, cleft lip, cleft palate, arching eyebrows, finger anomalies, postnatal growth deficiency, tooth anomalies, open mouth	•	•	•	•		•
Nager's Syndrome additional features include micrognathia, cleft or absent palate, external and middle-ear anomalies, hair on lateral cheek, downslanting palpebral fissures, absent lower eyelashes, atresia of external ear canal, high nasal bridge, preauricular tags	•	•				•
Oculo-Auriculo-Vertebral Spectrum additional features include facial asymmetry, spine anomalies, hypoplastic facial musculature, middle-ear anomalies, microtia, cleft palate, facial paresis, macrostomia, tongue anomalies, deep central dimple in chin, hypotelorism, iris coloboma, downslanting palpebralfissures	•	•	•	•		•
Townes' Syndrome additional features include microtia, facial asymmetry, commissural cleft, hemifacial microsomia, ear tags, auricular anomalies, hand anomalies					•	

	Speech	Resonance	Voice	Language	Hearing Sensorineural	Hearing Conductive
Treacher Collin Syndrome additional features include microtia, downslanting palpebral fissures, micrognathia, absent zygomas, cleft palate, flat frontonasal angle, lower lid coloboma, absent lower eyelashes, malformed auricles, low set ears, projection of scalp hair on to lateral cheek, molar hypoplasia, mandibular hypoplasia, iris coloboma	•	•				•
Wildervanck's Syndrome additional features include facial asymmetry, eye motility disorder, nystagmus, epibulbar dermoids, short neck, low hairline	•	•	•	•	•	•
4p- additional features include microcephaly, hypertelorism, ptosis, iris coloboma, broad hooked nose, micrognathia, hypotonia, strabismus, epicanthal folds, downturned corners of mouth, short upper lip and philtrum, absent earlobes, low posterior hairline, profound mental retardation	•	•	•	•		•
5p-/Cri-du-Chat Syndrome additional features include small stature, hypotonia, microcephaly, hypertelorism, epicanthal folds, downslanting palpebral fissures, facial asymmetry, strabismus, posteriorly rotated ears, low set ears, slow growth, cat-like cry, mental deficiency	•	•	•	•		•

Cup-Shaped Ears

	Speech	Resonance	Voice	Language	Hearing Sensorineural	Hearing Conductive
Blepharonasofacial Syndrome additional features include telecanthus, broad nasal root, cognitive impairment, midface hypoplasia, hyperextensible joints, hypertelorism	•		•			
Fraser's Syndrome additional features include syndactyly, small and abnormal genitals, scalp hair on forehead, cognitive impairment, cryptophthalmos, broad nose with depressed bridge, hypoplastic nares, hypertelorism	•		•	•		

Syndromes With Eye Anomalies
Eye Position
Hypotelorism

	Speech	Resonance	Voice	Language	Hearing Sensorineural	Hearing Conductive
Cockayne's Syndrome additional features include microcephaly, progressive cognitive impairment, central hearing impairment, optic atrophy, retinal pigmentation anomalies, nystagmus, profound postnatal growth deficiency, dental abnormalities, ataxia, dysarthic speech, seizures, loss of adipose tissue	•	•	•	•	•	
Frontonasal Dysplasia Sequence additional features include hypertelorism, cleft lip, strabismus, prominent forehead, broad nasal bridge, small mandible, flexion defects of fingers, coarse facies, partial anodontia, widow's peak	•	•		•	•	•
Hallermann-Streiff Syndrome additional features include short stature, micrognathia, small face, thin small pointed nose, nystagmus, sparse scalp hair and eyelashes, frontal and parietal bossing, cataracts, hypoplastic teeth, microphthalmia, blue sclera, alopecia, iris coloboma, microstomia, downslanting palpebral fissures, delayed closure of fontanels	•	•	•			
Holoprosencephaly additional features include absent bipolar development of brain, absence of olfactory bulbs and tracts, microcephaly, anosmia, cleft lip or cleft palate, single central incisor	•	•		•		•
Oculo-Auriculo-Vertebral Spectrum additional features include facial asymmetry, spine anomalies, hypoplastic facial musculature, middle-ear anomalies, microtia, cleft palate, facial paresis, macrostomia, preauricular tags and pits, tongue anomalies, deep central dimple in chin iris coloboma, downslanting palpebral fissures	•	•	•	•		•
Oculo-Dento-Digital Syndrome additional features include microphthalmia, small corneas, short palpebral fissures, epicanthal folds, small nares, sparse hair with abnormal texture, broad lower jaw, alopecia, enamel hypoplasia, syndactyly of fourth and fifth fingers	•				•	

	Speech	Resonance	Voice	Language	Hearing Sensorineural	Conductive
Opitz's Syndrome additional features include cleft palate, cleft lip, upward or downward slanting palpebral fissures, ocular hypertelorism, broad nasal bridge, short neck, cryptorchidism, hypospadias, widow's peak, posterior rotation of auricle, mild-to-moderate mental retardation	•	•	•	•		•
Trisomy 21/Down's Syndrome additional features include upslanted palpebral fissures, short stature, hypotonia, mental retardation, strabismus, short neck, macroglossia, midline parital hair whorl, low posterior hairline, late closure of fontanels, small nose, low nasal bridge, inner epicanthal folds, brushfield spots in iris, hypertelorism, nystagmus, cardiac anomalies, ear anomalies, protruding ears, microtia	•	•	•	•		•
Turner's Syndrome additional features include short stature, webbed neck, failure of puberty to occur, short neck, low posterior hairline, narrow maxilla, inner canthal folds, downslanting palpebral fissures, obesity, anomalous auricles, narrow palate, excessive pigmented nevi, blue sclera, iris coloboma			•			•
William's Syndrome additional features include short stature, hypercalcemia, macrostomia, hypertension, hyperopia, short palpebral fissures, cognitive problems, full lips, hoarse voice, depressed nasal bridge, epicanthal folds, mild microcephaly, medial eyebrow flare, blue eyes, stellate pattern to iris, hyperacusis	•			•		
Wolf-Hirschhorn Syndrome/ Chromosome 4p Syndrome additional features include microcephaly, cranial asymmetry, ear anomalies, ocular hypertelorism, short philtrum, cleft lip, cleft palate, strabismus, downslanting palpebral fissures, short hooked nose, iris coloboma, ptosis, nystagmus	•		•	•		

	Speech	Resonance	Voice	Language	Hearing Sensorineural	Conductive
18p- additional features include small stature, microcephaly, short neck, retrognathia, deep central dimple in chin, macrostomia, downturned corners of mouth	•	•		•		

Hypertelorism

	Speech	Resonance	Voice	Language	Hearing Sensorineural	Conductive
Aarskog-Scott Syndrome additional features include hypodontia, brachydactyly, short stature, small nose, broad philtrum, crease below the lower lip, maxillary hypoplasia, broad central upper incisors, cognitive impairment, ADD, ptosis of eyelids, downslanting palpebral fissures, widow's peak	•	•		•		
Apert's Syndrome additional features include syndactyly, hydrocephalus, cognitive impairment, high forehead, large fontanels with late closure, strabismus, small nose, narrow palate with median groove, downslanting palpebral fissures, occasional cleft palate, irregular craniosynostosis, fusion of cervical vertebrae, flat facies, shallow orbits, nystagmus, short anterio-posterior craniofacial diameter	•	•	•	•		•
Bixler's Syndrome additional features include short stature, cleft lip, cleft palate, heart anomalies, frontal bossing, craniosynostosis, microtia, depressed nasal bridge, dysplastic ears, anomalous ossicles, cognitive impairment	•	•		•		•
Blepharonasofacial Syndrome additional features include telecanthus, broad nasal root, cognitive impairment, midface hypoplasia, hyperextensible joints, cup-shaped ears	•			•		
Carpenter's Syndrome additional features include polydactyly, cognitive impairment, heart anomalies, lateral displacement of inner canthi, inner canthal folds, craniosynostosis, small stature, flat nasal bridge, optic atrophy, obesity, variable synostosis, brachydactyly of hands, low set malformed ears, high arched palate, large fontanels	•	•		•		

	Speech	Resonance	Voice	Language	Hearing Sensorineural	Conductive
Cat Eye Syndrome additional features include iris coloboma, cognitive impairment, short stature, anal anomalies, hernias, downslanting palpebral fissures, micrognathia, preauricular pits and tags, cardiac defects	•	•		•		•
Coffin-Lowry/Coffin-Siris Syndrome additional features include coarse facies, small stature, hypotonia, puffy hands, hypodontia, full lips, downslanting palpebral fissures, maxillary hypoplasia, short broad nose, prominent ears, growth deficiency, macrostomia, tapering fingers, coarse appearance	•			•		
Crouzon's Syndrome additional features include macrocephaly, maxillary hypoplasia, frontal bossing, upslanting palpebral fissures, low set ears, hypoplastic maxilla, ocular proptosis, nystagmus, mental retardation, iris coloboma, strabismus, optic atrophy, inverted V shape to palate, craniosynostosis	•	•				•
Fetal Alcohol Syndrome additional features include growth deficiency, low birth weight, microcephaly, short palpebral fissures, short nose, cleft palate, maxillary hypoplasia, smooth philtrum with thin and smooth upper lip, cognitive impairment, joint anomalies, protruding ears, numerous hair whorls	•	•	•	•		•
Fetal Hydantoin Syndrome additional features include growth deficiency, cleft palate, cleft lip, short nose, flat philtrum, low anterior hairline, hypoplastic distal phalanges, hirsutism, wide anterior fontanel, broad nasal bridge, bowed upper lip, cognitive impairment, short neck, abnormal palmar crease, coarse hair, low posterior hairline, upslanting palpebral fissures, delayed closure of fontanels	•	•		•		•
Fraser's Syndrome additional features include syndactyly, small and abnormal genitals, scalp hair on forehead, cognitive impairment, cryptophthalmos, broad nose with depressed bridge, hypoplastic nares, cup-shaped ears	•		•	•		

	Speech	Resonance	Voice	Language	Hearing Sensorineural	Conductive
Freeman-Sheldon Syndrome additional features include mask-like face, micrognathia, ulnar deviation of fingers, limited oral opening, broad nasal bridge, telecanthus, strabismus, small nose, small tongue, epicanthal folds, small mouth, deep set eyes, joint anomalies, downslanting palpebral fissures	•	•				•
Frontonasal Dysplasia Sequence additional features include cleft lip, strabismus, prominent forehead, broad nasal bridge, small mandible, flexion defects of fingers, coarse facies, partial anodontia, widow's peak, hypotelorism	•	•		•	•	•
LEOPARD Syndrome additional features include multiple lentigines, electrocardiographic conduct abnormalities, pulmonic stenosis, abnormal genitalia, mild growth deficiency, protruding ears, cryptorchidism, nystagmus	•	•		•	•	
Marinesco-Sjögren Syndrome additional features include microcephaly, small stature, cognitive impairment, ataxia, cataracts, ichthyosis, nystagmus	•	•		•		
Noonan's Syndrome additional features include short stature, ptosis of eyelids, low posterior hairline, webbed neck, short neck, downslanting eyes, cardiac defect, epicanthal folds, myopia, nystagmus, strabismus, malocclusion, cognitive impairment, wide mouth, prominent upper lip, retrognathia, low set ears, downslanting palpebral fissures	•	•	•	•	•	•
Opitz's Syndrome additional features include cleft palate, cleft lip, upward or downward slanting palpebral fissures, ocular broad nasal bridge, short neck, cryptorchidism, hypospadias, widow's peak, posterior rotation of auricle, mild-to-moderate mental retardation, hypotelorism	•	•	•	•		•

	Speech	Resonance	Voice	Language	Hearing Sensorineural	Hearing Conductive
Oto-Palato-Digital Syndrome, Type I additional features include downslanting eyes, small stature, cleft soft palate, micrognathia, microstomia, frontal prominence, large fontanels with delayed closure, low set ears, steep naso-basal angulation, small nose, cognitive impairment, hypoplastic facial bones, broad distal phalanges, downslanting palpebral fissures, upslanting palpebral fissures	•	•	•	•		•
Robinow's Syndrome additional features include macrocephaly, cleft palate, brachydactyly, vertebral and skeletal anomalies, short forearms, short stature, prominent eyes, small upturned nose, large anterior fontanel, long philtrum, downslanting palpebral fissures, triangular mouth with downturned angles, micrognathia, crowded teeth, posteriorly rotated ears, alopecia, microstomia, delayed closure of fontanels	•	•				•
Rubinstein-Taybi Syndrome additional features include beaked nose with nasal septum, cognitive impairment, short stature, downslanting palpebral fissures, hypoplastic maxilla, epicanthal folds, frontal hair upsweep, small mouth, deviated nasal septum, low set and malformed auricles, low posterior-anterior hairline, heavy eyebrows, broad great toes, long eyelashes, epicanthal folds, strabismus, hirsutism, iris coloboma	•		•	•		
Saethre-Chotzen Syndrome additional features include acrocephaly, syndactyly of hands and feet, brachycephaly, high forehead, maxillary hypoplasia, deviated nasal septum, small ears, ptosis of eyelid, craniosynostosis, large fontanels with delayed closure						•
Sotos' Syndrome additional features include large size at birth, large stature, large hands and feet, cognitive impairment, hypotonia, macrocephaly, prominent forehead, large ears, downslanting palpebral fissures, high narrow palate, premature eruption of teeth, sparse hair, thin brittle fingernails	•		•	•		

	Speech	Resonance	Voice	Language	Hearing Sensorineural	Conductive
Trisomy 21/Down's Syndrome additional features include upslanted palpebral fissures, short stature, hypotonia, mental retardation, strabismus, short neck, macroglossia, midline parital hair whorl, low posterior hairline, late closure of fontanels, small nose, low nasal bridge, inner epicanthal folds, brushfield spots in iris, hypotelorism, nystagmus, cardiac anomalies, ear anomalies, protruding ears, microtia	•	•	•	•		•
Weaver's Syndrome additional features include thin hair, accelerated growth, skeletal anomalies, large fontanels, macrocephaly, macrostomia, developmental delay, large protruding ears, camptodactyly, foot deformities, epicanthal folds, long philtrum, broad forehead, downslanting palpebral fissures, coarse and low-pitched voice, progressive spasticity, strabismus	•		•	•		
Wolf-Hirschhorn Syndrome/ Chomosome 4p Syndrome additional features include microcephaly, cranial asymmetry, ear anomalies, hypotelorism, short philtrum, cleft lip, cleft palate, strabismus, downslanting palpebral fissures, short hooked nose, iris coloboma, ptosis, nystagmus	•		•	•		
4p- additional features include microcephaly, ptosis, iris coloboma, broad hooked nose, micrognathia, hypotonia, strabismus, epicanthal folds, downturned corners of mouth, short upper lip and philtrum, preauricular tags and pits, absent earlobes, low posterior hairline, profound mental retardation	•	•	•	•		•
5q+ additional features include microcephaly, large ears, downslanting eyes, strabismus, micrognathia, cognitive deficiency	•			•		
8q+ additional features include cognitive deficiency, short nose, abnormal skull shape, low set ears	•	•		•		

	Speech	Resonance	Voice	Language	Hearing Sensorineural	Hearing Conductive
9p- additional features include cognitive deficiency, microstomia, micrognathia, ear lobe anomalies, craniosynostosis, short neck, upslanting palpebral fissures, prominent eyes, higher arched eyebrows, depressed nasal bridge, long philtrum, long middle phalanges of fingers	•	•		•		•
13q- additional features include microcephaly, severe cognitive deficiency, short neck, webbed neck, broad nasal root, frontal bossing, ptosis, colobomata, epicanthal folds, large slanting ears, microphthalmia	•		•	•		

Eye movement anomalies
Nystagmus

	Speech	Resonance	Voice	Language	Hearing Sensorineural	Hearing Conductive
Apert's Syndrome additional features include syndactyly, hydrocephalus, cognitive impairment, hypertelorism, high forehead, large fontanels with late closure, strabismus, small nose, narrow palate with median groove, downslanting palpebral fissures, occasional cleft palate, irregular craniosynostosis, fusion of cervical vertebrae, flat facies, shallow orbits, short anterio-posterior craniofacial diameter	•	•	•	•		•
Basal-Cell Nevus Syndrome additional features include macrocephaly, scoliosis, strabismus, basal cell carcinomas, frontoparietal bossing, broad nasal bridge, prognathism, occasional cognitive impairment, sloping narrow shoulders, vertebral anomalies, heavy fused eyebrows, misshapen carious teeth, epidermal cysts, nevi	•	•		•		
Bloch-Sulzberger Syndrome/ Incontinentia Pigmenti Syndrome additional features include strabismus, hypodontia, central nervous system anomalies, alopecia, retinal detachment, cataracts, microcephaly, mental deficiency, coarse hair, sparse hair in early childhood, linear distribution of blisters along limbs and trunk, hyperpigmentation on lines of Blaschko	•			•		

	Speech	Resonance	Voice	Language	Hearing Sensorineural	Conductive
Cardio-Facio-Cutaneous Syndrome additional features include large forehead, sparse curly scalp hair, depressed nasal root, short neck, ptosis, small stature, hypotonia, cardiac anomalies, posteriorly rotated ears, strabismus, mild-to-moderate mental retardation, shallow orbital ridges, brain anomalies, relative macrocephaly, downslanting palpebral fissures	•	•	•	•		
CHARGE Syndrome additional features include iris coloboma, heart anomalies, choanal atresia, growth retardation, ear anomalies, genital anomalies, micrognathia, cleft lip, facial palsy, mental deficiency, short neck	•	•	•	•	•	•
Crouzon's Syndrome additional features include macrocephaly, maxillary hypoplasia, hypertelorism, frontal bossing, upslanting palpebral fissures, low set ears, hypoplastic maxilla, ocular proptosis, mental retardation, iris coloboma, strabismus, optic atrophy, inverted V shape to palate, craniosynostosis	•	•				•
DeLange's Syndrome additional features include short stature, limb reduction, depressed nasal bridge, microcephaly, hypertonia, cleft palate, low anterior hairline, thin upper lip, short neck, micrognathia, long curly eyelashes, downturned corners of mouth, high arched palate, mental retardation, bushy eyebrows, hirsutism, clinodactyly of fifth fingers, simian creases, blue sclera, downslanting palpebral fissures	•	•	•	•	•	•
Fanconi's Pancytopenia Syndrome additional features include short stature, microcephaly, small or absent thumbs, renal anomalies, strabismus, hypoplastic radii, cognitive impairment, eye anomalies, hyperpigmentation	•			•		•

	Speech	Resonance	Voice	Language	Hearing Sensorineural	Conductive
Goltz's Syndrome additional features include microtia, downslanting palpebral fissures, micrognathia, absent zygomas, cleft palate, flat frontonasal angle, lower lid coloboma, absent lower eyelashes, malformed auricles, low set ears, projection of scalp hair on to lateral cheek, molar hypoplasia, mandibular hypoplasia, iris coloboma	•	•				•
Hallermann-Streiff Syndrome additional features include facial asymmetry, eye motility disorder, nystagmus, epibulbar dermoids, short neck, low hairline	•	•	•	•	•	•
4p- additional features include microcephaly, hypertelorism, ptosis, iris coloboma, broad hooked nose, micrognathia, hypotonia, strabismus, epicanthal folds, downturned corners **Hurler's Syndrome** absent earlobes, low posterior hairline, profound mental retardation	•	•	•	•		•
5p-/Cri-du-Chat Syndrome additional features include small stature, hypotonia, microcephaly, hypertelorism, epicanthal folds, downslanting palpebral fissures, facial asymmetry, strabismus, posteriorly rotated ears, low set ears, slow growth, **LEOPARD Syndrome**	•	•	•	•		•

ip-Shaped Ears

	Speech	Resonance	Voice	Language	Hearing Sensorineural	Conductive
Blepharonasofacial Syndrome additional features include telecanthus, broad nasal root, cognitive impairment, midface **Louis-Bar's Syndrome** additional features include athetosis,	•			•		
Fraser's Syndrome additional features include syndactyly, small and abnormal genitals, scalp hair on forehead, **Lowe's Syndrome** cryptophthalmos, broad nose with depressed bridge, hypoplastic nares, hypertelorism	•		•	•		

	Speech	Resonance	Voice	Language	Hearing Sensorineural	Hearing Conductive
Marfan's Syndrome additional features include tall stature, abnormal skeletal growth pattern, hyperextensible joints, hypotonia, myopia, retinal detachment, blue sclera, iris coloboma, arachnodactyly, narrow facies with narrow palate, hernias	•	•				
Marinesco-Sjögren Syndrome additional features include microcephaly, small stature, cognitive impairment, ataxia, cataracts, ichthyosis, hypertelorism	•	•		•		
Noonan's Syndrome additional features include short stature, ptosis of eyelids, low posterior hairline, webbed neck, short neck, downslanting eyes, cardiac defect, epicanthal folds, hypertelorism, myopia, strabismus, malocclusion, cognitive impairment, wide mouth, prominent upper lip, retrognathia, low set ears, downslanting palpebral fissures	•	•	•	•	•	•
Seckel Syndrome additional features include severe short stature, microcephaly, cognitive impairment, micrognathia, receding forehead, prominent nose, low set ears, absent ear lobe, downslanting palpebral fissures, simian crease, digital anomalies	•		•	•		
Trisomy 21/Down's Syndrome additional features include upslanted palpebral fissures, short stature, hypotonia, mental retardation, strabismus, short neck, macroglossia, midline parital hair whorl, low posterior hairline, late closure of fontanels, small nose, low nasal bridge, inner epicanthal folds, brushfield spots in iris, hypotelorism, hypertelorism, cardiac anomalies, ear anomalies, protruding ears, microtia	•	•	•	•		•

	Speech	Resonance	Voice	Language	Hearing Sensorineural	Conductive
Velo-Cardio-Facial Syndrome/ DiGeorge's Sequence additional features include short stature, microcephaly, cleft palate, long nose, prominent nose, puffy upper eyelids, squared nasal root, protruding ears, absent earlobes, microtia, vertical maxillary excess, long face, narrow palpebral fissures, downslanting palpebral fissures, abundant scalp hair, slender hands and feet, learning disabilities, heart anomalies, mild intellectual impairment	•	•	•	•	•	•
Werner's Syndrome additional features include short stature, small hands and feet, beaked nose, premature aging, hyperkeratosis, skin ulcerations, alopecia, sparse gray hair, loss of subcutaneous fat, premature loss of teeth, osteoporosis, hypogonadism, cataracts, retinal degeneration, blue sclera	•			•		
Wildervanck's Syndrome additional features include facial asymmetry, eye motility disorder, epibulbar dermoids, short neck, low hairline, preauricular tags and pits	•	•	•	•	•	•
Wolf-Hirschhorn Syndrome/ Chromosome 4p Syndrome additional features include microcephaly, cranial asymmetry, ear anomalies, ocular hypertelorism, hypotelorism, short philtrum, cleft lip, cleft palate, strabismus, downslanting palpebral fissures, short hooked nose, iris coloboma, ptosis	•		•	•		

Downslanting Palpebral Fissures
(Downward displacement of temporal canthus)

	Speech	Resonance	Voice	Language	Hearing Sensorineural	Conductive
Aarskog-Scott Syndrome additional features include hypodontia, brachydactyly, short stature, small nose, broad philtrum, crease below the lower lip, maxillary hypoplasia, broad central upper incisors, cognitive impairment, ADD, ptosis of eyelids, widow's peak, hypertelorism	•	•	•			

	Speech	Resonance	Voice	Language	Hearing Sensorineural	Conductive
Apert's Syndrome additional features include syndactyly, hydrocephalus, cognitive impairment, hypertelorism, high forehead, large fontanels with late closure, strabismus, small nose, narrow palate with median groove, occasional cleft palate, irregular craniosynostosis, fusion of cervical vertebrae, flat facies, shallow orbits, nystagmus, short anterio-posterior craniofacial diameter	•	•	•	•		•
Cardio-Facio-Cutaneous Syndrome additional features include large forehead, sparse curly scalp hair, depressed nasal root, short neck, ptosis, small stature, hypotonia, cardiac anomalies, posteriorly rotated ears, nystagmus, strabismus, mild-to-moderate mental retardation, shallow orbital ridges, brain anomalies, relative macrocephaly	•	•	•	•		
Cat Eye Syndrome additional features include iris coloboma, hypertelorism, cognitive impairment, short stature, anal anomalies, hernias, micrognathia, preauricular pits and tags, cardiac defects	•	•		•		•
Coffin-Lowry/Coffin-Siris Syndrome additional features include coarse facies, small stature, hypotonia, puffy hands, hypodontia, full lips, maxillary hypoplasia, short broad nose, prominent ears, growth deficiency, macrostomia, tapering fingers, coarse appearance, hypertelorism	•			•		
Cohen's Syndrome additional features include short stature, cognitive impairment, hypotonia, obesity, scoliosis, narrow face, high nasal root, downslanting eyes, microcephaly, decreased visual acuity, narrow hands and feet, simian creases, hyperextensible joints, delayed puberty, prominent maxillary incisors, high narrow palate, large ears	•			•		

	Speech	Resonance	Voice	Language	Hearing Sensorineural	Conductive
DeLange's Syndrome additional features include short stature, limb reduction, depressed nasal bridge, microcephaly, hypertonia, cleft palate, low anterior hairline, thin upper lip, short neck, micrognathia, long curly eyelashes, downturned corners of mouth, high arched palate, mental retardation, bushy eyebrows, hirsutism, clinodactyly of fifth fingers, simian creases, blue sclera, nystagmus	•	•	•	•	•	•
Freeman-Sheldon Syndrome additional features include mask-like face, micrognathia, ulnar deviation of fingers, limited oral opening, broad nasal bridge, telecanthus, strabismus, small nose, small tongue, epicanthal folds, small mouth, deep set eyes, joint anomalies, hypertelorism	•	•				•
Hallermann--Streiff Syndrome additional features include short stature, micrognathia, small face, thin small pointed nose, nystagmus, sparse scalp hair and eyelashes, frontal and parietal bossing, cataracts, hypoplastic teeth, microphthalmia, blue sclera, alopecia, hypotelorism, iris coloboma, microstomia, delayed closure of fontanels	•	•	•			
Möbius Syndrome additional features include small mouth, micrognathia, hypoglossia, cleft palate, broad nose, telecanthus, facial asymmetry, hypodontia, high nasal bridge	•	•		•		
Nager's Syndrome additional features include micrognathia, cleft or absent palate, external and middle-ear anomalies, hair on lateral cheek, absent lower eyelashes, atresia of external ear canal, high nasal bridge, preauricular tags	•	•				•
Noonan's Syndrome additional features include short stature, ptosis of eyelids, low posterior hairline, webbed neck, short neck, downslanting eyes, cardiac defect, epicanthal folds, hypertelorism, myopia, nystagmus, strabismus, malocclusion, cognitive impairment, wide mouth, prominent upper lip, retrognathia, low set ears	•	•	•	•	•	•

	Speech	Resonance	Voice	Language	Hearing Sensorineural	Hearing Conductive
Oculo-Auriculo-Vertebral Spectrum additional features include facial asymmetry, spine anomalies, hypoplastic facial musculature, middle-ear anomalies, microtia, cleft palate, facial paresis, macrostomia, preauricular tags and pits, tongue anomalies, deep central dimple in chin, hypotelorism, iris coloboma	•	•	•	•		•
Oto-Palato-Digital Syndrome, Type I additional features include hypertelorism, downslanting eyes, small stature, cleft soft palate, micrognathia, microstomia, frontal prominence, large fontanels with delayed closure, low set ears, steep naso-basal angulation, small nose, cognitive impairment, hypoplastic facial bones, broad distal phalanges, upslanting palpebral fissures	•	•	•	•		•
Robinow's Syndrome additional features include hypertelorism, macrocephaly, cleft palate, brachydactyly, vertebral and skeletal anomalies, short forearms, short stature, prominent eyes, small upturned nose, large anterior fontanel, long philtrum, triangular mouth with downturned angles, micrognathia, crowded teeth, posteriorly rotated ears, alopecia, microstomia, delayed closure of fontanels	•	•				•
Rubinstein-Taybi Syndrome additional features include beaked nose with nasal septum, hypertelorism, cognitive impairment, short stature, hypoplastic maxilla, epicanthal folds, frontal hair upsweep, small mouth, deviated nasal septum, low set and malformed auricles, low posterior-anterior hairline, heavy eyebrows, broad great toes, long eyelashes, epicanthal folds, strabismus, hirsutism, iris coloboma	•		•	•		
Seckel Syndrome additional features include severe short stature, microcephaly, nystagmus, cognitive impairment, micrognathia, receding forehead, prominent nose, low set ears, absent ear lobe simian crease, digital anomalies	•		•	•		

	Speech	Resonance	Voice	Language	Hearing Sensorineural	Hearing Conductive
Sotos' Syndrome additional features include large size at birth, large stature, large hands and feet, cognitive impairment, hypotonia, macrocephaly, prominent forehead, large ears, hypertelorism, high narrow palate, premature eruption of teeth, sparse hair, thin brittle fingernails	•		•	•		
Treacher Collins Syndrome additional features include microtia, micrognathia, absent zygomas, cleft palate, flat frontonasal angle, lower lid coloboma, absent lower eyelashes, malformed auricles, low set ears, preauricular tags and pits, projection of scalp hair on to lateral cheek, molar hypoplasia, mandibular hypoplasia, iris coloboma	•	•				•
Turner's Syndrome additional features include short stature, webbed neck, failure of puberty to occur, short neck, low posterior hairline, narrow maxilla, inner canthal folds, obesity, anomalous auricles, narrow palate, excessive pigmented nevi, blue sclera, iris coloboma, hypotelorism			•			•
Velo-Cardio-Facial Syndrome/ DiGeorge's Sequence additional features include short stature, microcephaly, cleft palate, long nose, prominent nose, puffy upper eyelids, nystagmus, squared nasal root, protruding ears, absent earlobes, microtia, vertical maxillary excess, long face, narrow palpebral fissures, abundant scalp hair, slender hands and feet, learning disabilities, heart anomalies, mild intellectual impairment	•	•	•	•	•	•
Weaver's Syndrome additional features include thin hair, accelerated growth, skeletal anomalies, large fontanels, macrocephaly, macrostomia, ocular hypertelorism, developmental delay, large protruding ears, camptodactyly, foot deformities, epicanthal folds, long philtrum, broad forehead, coarse and low-pitched voice, progressive spasticity, strabismus	•		•	•		

	Speech	Resonance	Voice	Language	Hearing Sensorineural	Conductive
Wolf-Hirschhorn Syndrome/ Chromosome 4p Syndrome additional features include microcephaly, cranial asymmetry, ear anomalies, ocular hypertelorism, hypotelorism, short philtrum, cleft lip, cleft palate, strabismus, short hooked nose, iris coloboma, ptosis, nystagmus	•		•	•		
5p-/Cri-du-Chat Syndrome additional features include small stature, hypotonia, microcephaly, hypertelorism, epicanthal folds, facial asymmetry, strabismus, preauricular tags and pits, posteriorly rotated ears, low set ears, slow growth, cat-like cry, mental deficiency	•	•	•	•		•

Upslanting Palpebral Fissures
(Temporal canthus is higher than nasal canthus)

	Speech	Resonance	Voice	Language	Hearing Sensorineural	Conductive
Crouzon's Syndrome additional features include macrocephaly, maxillary hypoplasia, hypertelorism, frontal bossing, low set ears, hypoplastic maxilla, ocular proptosis, nystagmus, mental retardation, iris coloboma, strabismus, optic atrophy, inverted V shape to palate, craniosynostosis	•	•				•
Femoral-Facial Syndrome additional features include cleft palate, micrognathia, short nose, thin upper lip, ear anomalies	•	•				•
Fetal Hydantoin Syndrome additional features include growth deficiency, cleft palate, cleft lip, short nose, flat philtrum, low anterior hairline, hypoplastic distal phalanges, hirsutism, wide anterior fontanel, ocular hypertelorism, broad nasal bridge, bowed upper lip, cognitive impairment, short neck, abnormal palmar crease, coarse hair, low posterior hairline, delayed closure of fontanels	•	•		•		•
Klinefelter's Syndrome additional features include micropenis, cleft palate, obesity, elbow dysplasia, fifth finger clinodactyly, long limbs, tall slim stature, behavior problems, iris coloboma	•			•		

	Speech	Resonance	Voice	Language	Hearing Sensorineural	Conductive
Oto-Palato-Digital Syndrome, Type 1 additional features include hypertelorism, downslanting eyes, small stature, cleft soft palate, micrognathia, microstomia, frontal prominence, large fontanels with delayed closure, low set ears, steep naso-basal angulation, small nose, cognitive impairment, hypoplastic facial bones, broad distal phalanges, downslanting palpebral fissures	•	•	•	•		•
Prader-Willi Syndrome additional features include short stature, obesity, hypogonadism, hypotonia, small hands and feet, strabismus, blond hair, numerous hair whorls, blue eyes, fair skin, mental retardation, thin upper lip, excessive appetite, almond-shaped palpebral fissures	•	•	•	•		
Trisomy 21/Down's Syndrome additional features include short stature, hypotonia, mental retardation, strabismus, short neck, macroglossia, midline parital hair whorl, low posterior hairline, late closure of fontanels, small nose, low nasal bridge, inner epicanthal folds, brushfield spots in iris, hypotelorism, hypertelorism, nystagmus, cardiac anomalies, ear anomalies, protruding ears, microtia	•	•	•	•		•

Abnormal Color of Sclera
Blue Sclera

	Speech	Resonance	Voice	Language	Hearing Sensorineural	Conductive
DeLange's Syndrome additional features include short stature, limb reduction, depressed nasal bridge, microcephaly, hypertonia, cleft palate, low anterior hairline, thin upper lip, short neck, micrognathia, long curly eyelashes, downturned corners of mouth, high arched palate, mental retardation, bushy eyebrows, hirsutism, clinodactyly of fifth fingers, simian creases, nystagmus, downslanting palpebral fissures	•	•	•	•	•	•

	Speech	Resonance	Voice	Language	Hearing Sensorineural	Conductive
Hallermann-Streiff Syndrome additional features include short stature, micrognathia, small face, thin small pointed nose, nystagmus, sparse scalp hair and eyelashes, frontal and parietal bossing, cataracts, hypoplastic teeth, microphthalmia, alopecia, hypotelorism, iris coloboma, microstomia, downslanting palpebral fissures, delayed closure of fontanels	•	•	•			
Marfan's Syndrome additional features include tall stature, abnormal skeletal growth pattern, hyperextensible joints, hypotonia, myopia, retinal detachment, nystagmus, iris coloboma, arachnodactyly, narrow facies with narrow palate, hernias	•	•				
Osteogenesis Imperfecta Type I additional features include bone fragility, small face, small stature, late eruption and irregularly placed teeth, thin skin, otosclerosis, blue gray coloration of teeth, postnatal growth deficiency, triangular facial appearance, delayed closure of fontanels			•		•	•
Russell-Silver Syndrome additional features include small stature, body asymmetry, large cranium with small triangular face, downturned corners of mouth, late closure of anterior fontanel, micrognathia, hyperhidrosis, hypoglycemia, café au lait spots			•			
Turner's Syndrome additional features include short stature, webbed neck, failure of puberty to occur, short neck, low posterior hairline, narrow maxilla, inner canthal folds, downslanting palpebral fissures, obesity, anomalous auricles, narrow palate, excessive pigmented nevi, iris coloboma, hypotelorism			•			•
Werner's Syndrome additional features include short stature, small hands and feet, beaked nose, premature aging, hyperkeratosis, skin ulcerations, alopecia, sparse gray hair, loss of subcutaneous fat, premature loss of teeth, osteoporosis, hypogonadism, cataracts, retinal degeneration, nystagmus	•			•		

Iris Anomalies
Coloboma of Iris

	Speech	Resonance	Voice	Language	Hearing Sensorineural	Conductive
Aicardi's Syndrome additional features include microphthalmia, brain anomalies, cleft lip, cleft palate, microcephaly, partial to total agenesis of corpus collosum, cognitive impairment, optic nerve coloboma, spina bifida, rib anomalies	•	•		•		
Cat Eye Syndrome additional features include hypertelorism, cognitive impairment, short stature, anal anomalies, hernias, downslanting palpebral fissures, micrognathia, preauricular pits and tags, cardiac defects	•	•		•		•
CHARGE Syndrome additional features include heart anomalies, choanal atresia, growth retardation, ear anomalies, genital anomalies, nystagmus, micrognathia, cleft lip, facial palsy, mental deficiency, short neck	•	•	•	•	•	•
Crouzon's Syndrome additional features include macrocephaly, maxillary hypoplasia, hypertelorism, frontal bossing, upslanting palpebral fissures, low set ears, hypoplastic maxilla, ocular proptosis, nystagmus, mental retardation, strabismus, optic atrophy, inverted V shape to palate, craniosynostosis	•	•				•
Ellis-van Creveld Syndrome additional features include short stature, short limbs, anodontia, short upper lip, labial frenula, dysplastic nails, cleft palate, prominent nose, narrow palpebral fissures, abundant scalp hair, retruded mandible, neonatal teeth, short upper lip, polydactyly of fingers, short broad middle phalanges	•			•		
Goltz's Syndrome additional features include skin and nail anomalies, strabismus, small eyes, nystagmus, small stature, cognitive impairment, hypoplastic teeth, microphthalmus, syndactyly of fingers and/or toes, narrow nasal bridge, ear anomalies, sparse brittle hair, asymmetric hands and feet	•			•		

	Speech	Resonance	Voice	Language	Hearing Sensorineural	Conductive
Hallermann-Streiff Syndrome additional features include short stature, micrognathia, small face, thin small pointed nose, nystagmus, sparse scalp hair and eyelashes, frontal and parietal bossing,cataracts, hypoplastic teeth, microphthalmia, blue sclera, alopecia, hypotelorism, microstomia, downslanting palpebral fissures, delayed closure of fontanels	•	•	•			
Hurler's Syndrome additional features include short stature, dementia, coarse facial features, short neck, macroencephaly, corneal clouding, full lips, flared nostrils, low nasal bridge, inner epicanthal folds, retinal pigmentation, cognitive impairment, large tongue, small teeth, joint anomalies, heart anomalies, hirsutism, nystagmus	•	•	•	•	•	
Klinefelter's Syndrome additional features include micropenis, cleft palate, obesity, elbow dysplasia, fifth finger clinodactyly, long limbs, tall slim stature, behavior problems, upslanting palpebral fissures	•			•		
Marfan's Syndrome additional features include tall stature, abnormal skeletal growth pattern, hyperextensible joints, hypotonia, myopia, retinal detachment, nystagmus, blue sclera, arachnodactyly, narrow facies with narrow palate, hernias	•	•				
Oculo-Auriculo-Vertebral Spectrum additional features include facial asymmetry, spine anomalies, hypoplastic facial musculature, middle-ear anomalies, microtia, cleft palate, facial paresis, macrostomia, preauricular tags and pits, tongue anomalies, deep central dimple in chin, hypotelorism, downslanting palpebral fissures	•	•	•	•		•
Rieger's Syndrome additional features include hypodontia, maxillary deficiency, hernias, broad nasal bridge, thin upper lip, everted lower lip, glaucoma, optic atrophy, iris anomalies	•					

	Speech	Resonance	Voice	Language	Hearing Sensorineural	Conductive
Rubinstein-Taybi Syndrome additional features include beaked nose with nasal septum, hypertelorism, cognitive impairment, short stature, downslanting palpebral fissures, hypoplastic maxilla, epicanthal folds, frontal hair upsweep, small mouth, deviated nasal septum, low set and malformed auricles, low posterior-anterior hairline, heavy eyebrows, broad great toes, long eyelashes, epicanthal folds, strabismus, hirsutism	•		•	•		
Treacher Collins Syndrome additional features include microtia, downslanting palpebral fissures, micrognathia, absent zygomas, cleft palate, flat frontonasal angle, lower lid coloboma, absent lower eyelashes, malformed auricles, low set ears, preauricular tags and pits, projection of scalp hair onto lateral cheek, molar hypoplasia, mandibular hypoplasia	•	•				•
Turner's Syndrome additional features include short stature, webbed neck, failure of puberty to occur, short neck, low posterior hairline, narrow maxilla, inner canthal folds, downslanting palpebral fissures, obesity, anomalous auricles, narrow palate, excessive pigmented nevi, blue sclera, hypotelorism			•			•
Wolf-Hirschhorn Syndrome/ Chromosome 4p Syndrome additional features include microcephaly, cranial asymmetry, ear anomalies, ocular hypertelorism, hypotelorism, short philtrum, cleft lip, cleft palate, strabismus, downslanting palpebral fissures, short hooked nose, ptosis, nystagmus	•		•	•		
4p- additional features include microcephaly, hypertelorism, ptosis, broad hooked nose, micrognathia, hypotonia, strabismus, epicanthal folds, downturned corners of mouth, short upper lip and philtrum, preauricular tags and pits, absent earlobes, low posterior hairline, profound mental retardation	•	•	•	•		•

	Speech	Resonance	Voice	Language	Hearing Sensorineural	Conductive
13q- additional features include microcephaly, severe cognitive deficiency, short neck, webbed neck, broad nasal root, frontal bossing, hypertelorism, ptosis, epicanthal folds, large slanting ears, microphthalmia	•		•	•		

Heterochromia

	Speech	Resonance	Voice	Language	Hearing Sensorineural	Conductive
Neurofibromatosis-Type I additional features include café au lait spots, cutaneous neurofibromas, skeletal anomalies, pigmented iris	•	•	•	•		
Neurofibromatosis-Type II additional features include bilateral acoustic neuromas, CNS tumors, pigmented iris, short stature, cutaneous neurofibromas, café au lait spots	•				•	
Neurofibromatosis-Type III additional features include CNS tumors, acoustic neuromas, macroencephaly, optic glioma, short stature, café au lait spots	•			•	•	
Waardenburg Syndrome, Type I additional features include partial albinism, pigmentary anomalies of hair, white forelock, hypopigmentation, broad and high nasal bridge, broad mandible, full lips, medial flare of eyebrows, short palpebral fissures					•	

Syndromes With Hair Anomalies

Alopecia

	Speech	Resonance	Voice	Language	Hearing Sensorineural	Hearing Conductive
Bloch-Sulzberger Syndrome/ Incontinentia Pigmenti Syndromes additional features include strabismus, hypodontia, central nervous system anomalies, retinal detachment, cataracts, microcephaly, mental deficiency, nystagmus, coarse hair, sparse hair in early childhood, linear distribution of blisters along limbs and trunk, hyperpigmentation on lines of Blaschko	•		•			
Clouston's Syndrome additional features include thickened skin on palms and feet, strabismus, short stature, hypoplastic nails, hyperpigmentation, deficient eyelashes and eyebrows	•		•			
Hallermann-Streiff Syndrome additional features include short stature, micrognathia, small face, thin small pointed nose, nystagmus, sparse scalp hair and eyelashes, frontal and parietal bossing, cataracts, hypoplastic teeth, microphthalmia, blue sclera, hypotelorism, iris coloboma, microstomia, downslanting palpebral fissures, delayed closure of fontanels	•	•	•			
Hypohidrotic Ectodermal Dysplasia Syndrome additional features include thin fair skin, hypopigmentation, sparse fine hair, silver hair, hypodontia, small nose, thin and wrinkled eyelids, hypoplastic sweat glands, conical anterior teeth, full forehead, low nasal bridge, full lips	•		•			
Oculo-Dento-Digital Syndrome additional features include microphthalmia, hypotelorism, small corneas, short palpebral fissures, epicanthal folds, small nares, sparse hair with abnormal texture, broad lower jaw, enamel hypoplasia, syndactyly of fourth and fifth fingers	•				•	

	Speech	Resonance	Voice	Language	Hearing Sensorineural	Conductive
Robinow's Syndrome additional features include hypertelorism, macrocephaly, cleft palate, brachydactyly, vertebral and skeletal anomalies, short forearms, short stature, prominent eyes, small upturned nose, large anterior fontanel, long philtrum, downslanting palpebral fissures, triangular mouth with downturned angles, micrognathia, crowded teeth, posteriorly rotated ears, microstomia, delayed closure of fontanels	•	•				•
Werner's Syndrome additional features include short stature, small hands and feet, beaked nose, premature aging, hyperkeratosis, skin ulcerations, sparse gray hair, loss of subcutaneous fat, premature loss of teeth, osteoporosis, hypogonadism, cataracts, retinal degeneration, blue sclera, nystagmus	•			•		

Hirsutism

	Speech	Resonance	Voice	Language	Hearing Sensorineural	Conductive
Berardinelli-Lipodystrophy Syndrome additional features include enlarged liver and heart, cognitive impairment, muscular hypertrophy, tall stature, coarse skin, large superficial veins, absence of facial subcutaneous fat, hypertrophic tonsils and adenoids, curly scalp hair, accelerated growth and maturation, enlarged hands and feet, hyperpigmentation	•	•		•		
DeLange's Syndrome additional features include short stature, limb reduction, depressed nasal bridge, microcephaly, hypertonia, cleft palate, low anterior hairline, thin upper lip, short neck, micrognathia, long curly eyelashes, downturned corners of mouth, high arched palate, mental retardation, bushy eyebrows, clinodactyly of fifth fingers, simian creases, blue sclera, nystagmus, downslanting palpebral fissures	•	•	•	•	•	•

	Speech	Resonance	Voice	Language	Hearing Sensorineural	Conductive
Fetal Hydantoin Syndrome additional features include growth deficiency, cleft palate, cleft lip, short nose, flat philtrum, low anterior hairline, hypoplastic distal phalanges, wide anterior fontanel, ocular hypertelorism, broad nasal bridge, bowed upper lip, cognitive impairment, short neck, abnormal palmar crease, coarse hair, low posterior hairline, upslanting palpebral fissures, delayed closure of fontanels	•	•		•		•
Hurler's Syndrome additional features include short stature, dementia, coarse facial features, short neck, macroencephaly, corneal clouding, full lips, flared nostrils, low nasal bridge, inner epicanthal folds, retinal pigmentation, cognitive impairment, large tongue, small teeth, joint anomalies, heart anomalies, nystagmus, iris coloboma	•	•	•	•	•	
Rubinstein-Taybi Syndrome additional features include beaked nose with nasal septum, hypertelorism, cognitive impairment, short stature, downslanting palpebral fissures, hypoplastic maxilla, epicanthal folds, frontal hair upsweep, small mouth, deviated nasal septum, low set and malformed auricles, low posterior-anterior hairline, heavy eyebrows, broad great toes, long eyelashes, epicanthal folds, strabismus, iris coloboma	•		•	•		
Scheie's Syndrome additional features include liver enlargement, mild facial coarsening, full lips, broad mouth, deep central dimple in chin, macrostomia, corneal clouding, short neck, prognathic mandible, joint limitations			•			•

Texture Sparse Hair	Speech	Resonance	Voice	Language	Hearing Sensorineural	Conductive
Bloch-Sulzberger Syndrome/ Incontinentia Pigmenti Syndrome additional features include strabismus, hypodontia, central nervous system anomalies, alopecia, retinal detachment, cataracts, microcephaly, mental deficiency, nystagmus, coarse hair, sparse hair in early childhood, linear distribution of blisters along limbs and trunk, hyperpigmentation on lines of Blaschko	•			•		
Cardio-Facio-Cutaneous Syndrome additional features include large forehead, sparse curly scalp hair, depressed nasal root, short neck, ptosis, small stature, hypotonia, cardiac anomalies, posteriorly rotated ears, nystagmus, strabismus, mild-to-moderate mental retardation, shallow orbital ridges, brain anomalies, relative macrocephaly, downslanting palpebral fissures	•	•	•	•		
Hallermann-Streiff Syndrome additional features include short stature, micrognathia, small face, thin small pointed nose, nystagmus, sparse scalp hair and eyelashes, frontal and parietal bossing, cataracts, hypoplastic teeth, microphthalmia, blue sclera, alopecia, hypotelorism, iris coloboma, microstomia, downslanting palpebral fissures, delayed closure of fontanels	•	•	•			
Hypohidrotic Ectodermal Dysplasia Syndrome additional features include thin fair skin, hypopigmentation, alopecia, sparse fine hair, silver hair, hypodontia, small nose, thin and wrinkled eyelids, hypoplastic sweat glands, conical anterior teeth, full forehead, low nasal bridge, full lips	•		•			
Oculo-Dento-Digital Syndrome additional features include microphthalmia, hypotelorism, small corneas, short palpebral fissures, epicanthal folds, small nares, sparse hair with abnormal texture, broad lower jaw, alopecia, enamel hypoplasia, syndactyly of fourth and fifth fingers	•				•	

	Speech	Resonance	Voice	Language	Hearing Sensorineural	Hearing Conductive
Soto's Syndrome additional features include large size at birth, large stature, large hands and feet, cognitive impairment, hypotonia, macrocephaly, prominent forehead, large ears, hypertelorism, downslanting palpebral fissures, high narrow palate, premature eruption of teeth, thin brittle fingernails	•		•	•		
Tricho-Rhino-Pharyngeal Syndrome, Type I additional features include long nose, small carious teeth, thin nails, short stature, prominent and long philtrum, narrow palate, horizontal groove on chin, malocclusion, mild growth deficiency, digital anomalies, large prominent ears	•		•			
Werner's Syndrome additional features include short stature, small hands and feet, beaked nose, premature aging, hyperkeratosis, skin ulcerations, alopecia, sparse gray hair, loss of subcutaneous fat, premature loss of teeth, osteoporosis, hypogonadism, cataracts, retinal degeneration, blue sclera, nystagmus	•			•		

Coarse Hair

	Speech	Resonance	Voice	Language	Hearing Sensorineural	Hearing Conductive
Bloch-Sulzberger Syndrome/ Incontinentia Pigmenti Syndrome additional features include strabismus, hypodontia, central nervous system anomalies, alopecia, retinal detachment, cataracts, microcephaly, mental deficiency, nystagmus, sparse hair in early childhood, linear distribution of blisters along limbs and trunk, hyperpigmentation on lines of Blaschko	•			•		
Fetal Hydantoin Syndrome additional features include growth deficiency, cleft palate, cleft lip, short nose, flat philtrum, low anterior hairline, hypoplastic distal phalanges, hirsutism, wide anterior fontanel, ocular hypertelorism, broad nasal bridge, bowed upper lip, cognitive impairment, short neck, abnormal palmar crease, low posterior hairline, upslanting palpebral fissures, delayed closure of fontanels	•	•		•		•

Thin Hair

	Speech	Resonance	Voice	Language	Hearing Sensorineural	Conductive
Weaver's Syndrome additional features include accelerated growth, skeletal anomalies, large fontanels, macrocephaly, macrostomia, ocular hypertelorism, developmental delay, large protruding ears, camptodactyly, foot deformities, epicanthal folds, long philtrum, broad forehead, downslanting palpebral fissures, coarse and low-pitched voice, progressive spasticity, strabismus	•		•	•		

Silver Hair

	Speech	Resonance	Voice	Language	Sensorineural	Conductive
Hypohidrotic Ectodermal Dysplasia Syndrome additional features include thin fair skin, hypopigmentation, alopecia, sparse fine hair, hypodontia, small nose, thin and wrinkled eyelids, hypoplastic sweat glands, conical anterior teeth, full forehead, low nasal bridge, full lips	•		•			

White Hair

	Speech	Resonance	Voice	Language	Sensorineural	Conductive
Piebaldness additional features include hyperpigmented borders between pigmented and unpigmented zones, hypopigmentation	•	•			•	
Waardenburg Syndrome, Type I additional features include heterochromia, partial albinism, pigmentary anomalies of hair, hypopigmentation, broad and high nasal bridge, broad mandible, full lips, medial flare of eyebrows, short palpebral fissures					•	

Abnormal Hair Placement
Low Posterior Hairline

	Speech	Resonance	Voice	Language	Sensorineural	Conductive
Fetal Hydantoin Syndrome additional features include growth deficiency, cleft palate, cleft lip, short nose, flat philtrum, low anterior hairline, hypoplastic distal phalanges, hirsutism, wide anterior fontanel, ocular hypertelorism, broad nasal bridge, bowed upper lip, cognitive impairment, short neck, abnormal palmar crease, coarse hair, upslanting palpebral fissures, delayed closure of fontanels	•	•		•		•

	Speech	Resonance	Voice	Language	Hearing Sensorineural	Hearing Conductive
Noonan's Syndrome additional features include short stature, ptosis of eyelids, webbed neck, short neck, downslanting eyes, cardiac defect, epicanthal folds, hypertelorism, myopia, nystagmus, strabismus, malocclusion, cognitive impairment, wide mouth, prominent upper lip, retrognathia, low set ears, downslanting palpebral fissures	•	•	•	•	•	•
Rubinstein-Taybi Syndrome additional features include beaked nose with nasal septum, hypertelorism, cognitive impairment, short stature, downslanting palpebral fissures, hypoplastic maxilla, epicanthal folds, frontal hair upsweep, small mouth, deviated nasal septum, low set and malformed auricles, low anterior hairline, heavy eyebrows, broad great toes, long eyelashes, epicanthal folds, strabismus, hirsutism, iris coloboma	•		•	•		
Trisomy 21/Down's Syndrome additional features include upslanted palpebral fissures, short stature, hypotonia, mental retardation, strabismus, short neck, macroglossia, midline parital hair whorl, late closure of fontanels, small nose, low nasal bridge, inner epicanthal folds, brushfield spots in iris, hypotelorism, hypertelorism, nystagmus, cardiac anomalies, ear anomalies, protruding ears, microtia	•	•	•	•		•
Turner's Syndrome additional features include short stature, webbed neck, failure of puberty to occur, short neck, narrow maxilla, inner canthal folds, downslanting palpebral fissures, obesity, anomalous auricles, narrow palate, excessive pigmented nevi, blue sclera, iris coloboma, hypotelorism			•			•
4p- additional features include microcephaly, hypertelorism, ptosis, iris coloboma, broad hooked nose, micrognathia, hypotonia, strabismus, epicanthal folds, downturned corners of mouth, short upper lip and philtrum, preauricular tags and pits, absent earlobes, profound mental retardation	•	•	•	•		•

Low Anterior Hairline	Speech	Resonance	Voice	Language	Hearing Sensorineural	Conductive
DeLange's Syndrome additional features include short stature, limb reduction, depressed nasal bridge, microcephaly, hypertonia, cleft palate, thin upper lip, short neck, micrognathia, long curly eyelashes, downturned corners of mouth, high arched palate, mental retardation, bushy eyebrows, hirsutism, clinodactyly of fifth fingers, simian creases, blue sclera, nystagmus, downslanting palpebral fissures	•	•	•	•	•	•
Fetal Hydantoin Syndrome additional features include growth deficiency, cleft palate, cleft lip, short nose, flat philtrum, hypoplastic distal phalanges, hirsutism, wide anterior fontanel, ocular hypertelorism, broad nasal bridge, bowed upper lip, cognitive impairment, short neck, abnormal palmar crease, coarse hair, low posterior hairline, upslanting palpebral fissures, delayed closure of fontanels	•	•		•		•
Rubinstein-Taybi Syndrome additional features include beaked nose with nasal septum, hypertelorism, cognitive impairment, short stature, downslanting palpebral fissures, hypoplastic maxilla, epicanthal folds, frontal hair upsweep, small mouth, deviated nasal septum, low set and malformed auricles, low posterior hairline, heavy eyebrows, broad great toes, long eyelashes, epicanthal folds, strabismus, hirsutism, iris coloboma	•		•	•		

Hair on Lateral Cheek

	Speech	Resonance	Voice	Language	Hearing Sensorineural	Conductive
Nager's Syndrome additional features include micrognathia, cleft or absent palate, external and middle-ear anomalies, downslanting palpebral fissures, absent lower eyelashes, atresia of external ear canal, high nasal bridge preauricular tags	•	•				•
Treacher Collins Syndrome additional features include microtia, downslanting palpebral fissures, micrognathia, absent zygomas, cleft palate, flat frontonasal angle, lower lid coloboma, absent lower eyelashes, malformed auricles, low set ears, preauricular tags and pits, molar hypoplasia, mandibular hypoplasia, iris coloboma	•	•				•

Growth Pattern of Hair
Numerous Hair Whorls

	Speech	Resonance	Voice	Language	Hearing Sensorineural	Conductive
Fetal Alcohol Syndrome additional features include growth deficiency, low birth weight, microcephaly, short palpebral fissures, short nose, cleft palate, maxillary hypoplasia, smooth philtrum with thin and smooth upper lip, cognitive impairment, joint anomalies, hypertelorism, protruding ears	•	•	•	•		•
Prader-Willi Syndrome additional features include short stature, obesity, hypogonadism, hypotonia, small hands and feet, strabismus, blond hair, blue eyes, fair skin, mental retardation, thin upper lip, excessive appetite, almond-shaped palpebral fissures, upslanting palpebral fissures	•	•	•	•		

Widow's Peak

	Speech	Resonance	Voice	Language	Hearing Sensorineural	Conductive
Aarskog-Scott Syndrome additional features include hypodontia, brachydactyly, short stature, small nose, broad philtrum, crease below the lower lip, maxillary hypoplasia, broad central upper incisors, cognitive impairment, ADD, ptosis of eyelids, downslanting palpebral fissures, hypertelorism	•	•		•		
Frontonasal Dysplasia Sequence additional features include hypertelorism, cleft lip, strabismus, prominent forehead, broad nasal bridge, small mandible, flexion defects of fingers, coarse facies, partial anodontia, hypotelorism	•	•		•	•	•
Opitz's Syndrome additional features include cleft palate, cleft lip, upward or downward slanting palpebral fissures, ocular hypertelorism, broad nasal bridge, short neck, cryptorchidism, hypospadias, posterior rotation of auricle, mild-to-moderate mental retardation, hypotelorism	•	•	•	•		•

Eyelashes
Long Eyelashes

	Speech	Resonance	Voice	Language	Hearing Sensorineural	Hearing Conductive
DeLange's Syndrome additional features include short stature, limb reduction, depressed nasal bridge, microcephaly, hypertonia, cleft palate, low anterior hairline, thin upper lip, short neck, micrognathia, curly eyelashes, downturned corners of mouth, high arched palate, mental retardation, bushy eyebrows, hirsutism, clinodactyly of fifth fingers, simian creases, blue sclera, nystagmus, downslanting palpebral fissures	•	•	•	•	•	•
Rubinstein-Taybi Syndrome additional features include beaked nose with nasal septum, hypertelorism, cognitive impairment, short stature, downslanting palpebral fissures, hypoplastic maxilla, epicanthal folds, frontal hair upsweep, small mouth, deviated nasal septum, low set and malformed auricles, low posterior-anterior hairline, heavy eyebrows, broad great toes, epicanthal folds, strabismus, hirsutism, iris coloboma	•		•	•		

Absent Lower Eyelashes

	Speech	Resonance	Voice	Language	Hearing Sensorineural	Hearing Conductive
Nager's Syndrome additional features include micrognathia, cleft or absent palate, external and middle-ear anomalies, hair on lateral cheek, downslanting palpebral fissures, atresia of external ear canal, high nasal bridge, preauricular tags	•	•				•
Treacher Collins Syndrome additional features include microtia, downslanted palpebral fissures, micrognathia, absent zygomas, cleft palate, flat frontonasal angle, lower lid coloboma, malformed auricles, low set ears, preauricular tags and pits, projection of scalp hair onto lateral cheek, molar hypoplasia, mandibular hypoplasia, iris coloboma	•	•				•

Sparse Eyelashes

	Speech	Resonance	Voice	Language	Hearing Sensorineural	Hearing Conductive
Hallermann-Streiff Syndrome additional features include short stature, micrognathia, small face, thin small pointed nose, nystagmus, sparse scalp hair, frontal and parietal bossing, cataracts, hypoplastic teeth, microphthalmia, blue sclera, alopecia, hypotelorism, iris coloboma, microstomia, downslanting palpebral fissures, delayed closure of fontanels	•	•	•			

Syndromes With Lip/Mouth Anomalies
Downturned Corners of Mouth

	Speech	Resonance	Voice	Language	Hearing Sensorineural	Conductive
DeLange's Syndrome additional features include short stature, limb reduction, depressed nasal bridge, microcephaly, hypertonia, cleft palate, low anterior hairline, thin upper lip, short neck, micrognathia, long curly eyelashes, high arched palate, mental retardation, bushy eyebrows, hirsutism, clinodactyly of fifth fingers, simian creases, blue sclera, nystagmus, downslanting palpebral fissures	•	•	•	•	•	•
Robinow's Syndrome additional features include hypertelorism, macrocephaly, cleft palate, brachydactyly, vertebral and skeletal anomalies, short forearms, short stature, prominent eyes, small upturned nose, large anterior fontanel, long philtrum, downslanting palpebral fissures, triangular mouth, micrognathia, crowded teeth, posteriorly rotated ears, alopecia, microstomia, delayed closure of fontanels	•	•				•
Russell-Silver Syndrome additional features include small stature, body asymmetry, large cranium with small triangular face, late closure of anterior fontanel, micrognathia, hyperhidrosis, hypoglycemia, blue sclera, café au lait spots			•			
4p- additional features include microcephaly, hypertelorism, ptosis, iris coloboma, broad hooked nose, micrognathia, hypotonia, strabismus, epicanthal folds, short upper lip and philtrum, preauricular tags and pits, absent earlobes, low posterior hairline, profound mental retardation	•	•	•	•		•
4q+ additional features include microcephaly, short stature, posteriorly rotated ears, low set ears, cleft palate, prominent forehead	•		•			•
6q+ additional features include microcephaly, short stature, cleft palate, prominent forehead, low set ears	•	•	•	•		•

	Speech	Resonance	Voice	Language	Hearing Sensorineural	Conductive
18p- additional features include small stature, microcephaly, short neck, hypotelorism, retrognathia, deep central dimple in chin, macrostomia	•	•		•		

Deep Central Dimple in Chin

	Speech	Resonance	Voice	Language	Hearing Sensorineural	Conductive
Morquio's Syndrome additional features include short stature, corneal clouding, joint and spine anomalies, short neck, macrostomia, short nose, widely spaced teeth, coarse facial features, thin enamel on teeth		•	•		•	•
Oculo-Auriculo-Vertebral Spectrum additional features include facial asymmetry, spine anomalies, hypoplastic facial musculature, middle-ear anomalies, microtia, cleft palate, facial paresis, macrostomia, preauricular tags and pits, tongue anomalies, hypotelorism, iris coloboma, downslanting palpebral fissures	•	•	•	•		•
Scheie's Syndrome additional features include liver enlargement, mild facial coarsening, full lips, broad mouth, macrostomia, corneal clouding, hirsutism, short neck, prognathic mandible, joint limitations			•			•
18p- additional features include small stature, microcephaly, short neck, hypotelorism, retrognathia, macrostomia, downturned corners of mouth	•	•		•		

Macrostomia

	Speech	Resonance	Voice	Language	Hearing Sensorineural	Conductive
Angelman's Syndrome additional features include microcephaly, ataxic arm movements, seizures, cognitive impairment, decreased pigmentation of iris and choroid, maxillary hypoplasia, widely spaced teeth, blond hair, pale blue eyes, optic atrophy, prognathic mandible, inappropriate laughter, absent speech, large fontanels	•					

	Speech	Resonance	Voice	Language	Hearing Sensorineural	Conductive
Morquio's Syndrome additional features include short stature, corneal clouding, joint and spine anomalies, short neck, hort nose, widely spaced teeth, coarse facial features, thin enamel on teeth, deep central dimple in chin		•	•		•	•
Oculo-Auriculo-Vertebral Spectrum additional features include facial asymmetry, spine anomalies, hypoplastic facial musculature, middle-ear anomalies, microtia, cleft palate, facial paresis, preauricular tags and pits, tongue anomalies, deep central dimple in chin, hypotelorism, iriscoloboma, downslanting palpebral fissures	•	•	•	•		•
Scheie's Syndrome additional features include liver enlargement, mild facial coarsening, full lips, broad mouth, deep central dimple in chin, corneal clouding, hirsutism, short neck, prognathic mandible, joint limitations			•			•
Weaver's Syndrome additional features include thin hair, accelerated growth, skeletal anomalies, large fontanels, macrocephaly, ocular hypertelorism, developmental delay, large protruding ears, camptodactyly, foot deformities, epicanthal folds, long philtrum, broad forehead, downslanting palpebral fissures, coarse and low-pitched voice, progressive spasticity, strabismus	•		•	•		
Williams' Syndrome additional features include short stature, hypercalcemia, hypertension, hyperopia, hypotelorism, short palpebral fissures, cognitive problems, full lips, hoarse voice, depressed nasal bridge, epicanthal folds, mild microcephaly, medial eyebrow flare, blue eyes, stellate pattern to iris, hyperacusis	•			•		
18p- additional features include small stature, microcephaly, short neck, hypotelorism, retrognathia, deep central dimple in chin, downturned corners of mouth	•	•		•		

Microstomia	Speech	Resonance	Voice	Language	Hearing Sensorineural	Conductive
Hallermann-Streiff Syndrome additional features include short stature, micrognathia, small face, thin small pointed nose, nystagmus, sparse scalp hair and eyelashes, frontal and parietal bossing, cataracts, hypoplastic teeth, microphthalmia, blue sclera, alopecia, hypotelorism, iris coloboma, downslanting palpebral fissures, delayed closure of fontanels	•	•	•			
Oto-Palato-Digital Syndrome, Type I additional features include hypertelorism, downslanting eyes, small stature, cleft soft palate, micrognathia, frontal prominence, large fontanels with delayed closure, low set ears, steep naso-basal angulation, small nose, cognitive impairment, hypoplastic facial bones, broad distal phalanges, downslanting palpebral fissures, upslanting palpebral fissures	•	•	•	•		•
Robinow's Syndrome additional features include hypertelorism, macrocephaly, cleft palate, brachydactyly, vertebral and skeletal anomalies, short forearms, short stature, prominent eyes, small upturned nose, large anterior fontanel, long philtrum, downslanting palpebral fissures, triangular mouth with downturned angles, micrognathia, crowded teeth, posteriorly rotated ears, alopecia, delayed closure of fontanels	•	•				•
9p- additional features include hypertelorism, cognitive deficiency, micrognathia, ear lobe anomalies, craniosynostosis, short neck, upslanting palpebral fissures, prominent eyes, higher arched eyebrows, depressed nasal bridge, long philtrum, long middle phalanges of fingers	•	•		•		•

Full Lips

	Speech	Resonance	Voice	Language	Hearing Sensorineural	Conductive
Coffin-Lowry/Coffin-Siris Syndrome additional features include coarse facies, small stature, hypotonia, puffy hands, hypodontia, downslanting palpebral fissures, maxillary hypoplasia, short broad nose, prominent ears, growth deficiency, macrostomia, tapering fingers, coarse appearance, hypertelorism	•			•		

	Speech	Resonance	Voice	Language	Hearing Sensorineural	Conductive
Hurler's Syndrome additional features include short stature, dementia, coarse facial features, short neck, macroencephaly, corneal clouding, flared nostrils, low nasal bridge, inner epicanthal folds, retinal pigmentation, cognitive impairment, large tongue, small teeth, joint anomalies, heart anomalies, hirsutism, nystagmus, iris coloboma	•	•	•	•	•	
Hypohidrotic Ectodermal Dysplasia Syndrome additional features include thin fair skin, hypopigmentation, alopecia, sparse fine hair, silver hair, hypodontia, small nose, thin and wrinkled eyelids, hypoplastic sweat glands, conical anterior teeth, full forehead, low nasal bridge	•		•			
Noonan's Syndrome additional features include short stature, ptosis of eyelids, low posterior hairline, webbed neck, short neck, downslanting eyes, cardiac defect, epicanthal folds, hypertelorism, myopia, nystagmus, strabismus, malocclusion, cognitive impairment, wide mouth, prominent upper lip, retrognathia, low set ears, downslanting palpebral fissures	•	•	•	•	•	•
Scheie's Syndrome additional features include liver enlargement, mild facial coarsening, broad mouth, deep central dimple in chin, macrostomia, corneal clouding, hirsutism, short neck, prognathic mandible, joint limitations			•			•
Waardenburg Syndrome, Type I additional features include heterochromia, partial albinism, pigmentary anomalies of hair, white forelock, hypopigmentation, broad and high nasal bridge, broad mandible, medial flare of eyebrows, short palpebral fissures					•	
Williams' Syndrome additional features include short stature, hypercalcemia, macrostomia, hypertension, hyperopia, hypotelorism, short palpebral fissures, cognitive problems, hoarse voice, depressed nasal bridge, epicanthal folds, mild microcephaly, medial eyebrow flare, blue eyes, stellate pattern to iris, hyperacusis	•			•		

Syndromes With Neck Anomalies

Webbed Neck

	Speech	Resonance	Voice	Language	Hearing Sensorineural	Hearing Conductive
Noonan's Syndrome additional features include short stature, ptosis of eyelids, low posterior hairline, short neck, downslanting eyes, cardiac defect, epicanthal folds, hypertelorism, myopia, nystagmus, strabismus, malocclusion, cognitive impairment, wide mouth, prominent upper lip, retrognathia, low set ears, downslanting palpebral fissures	•	•	•	•	•	•
Turner's Syndrome additional features include short stature, failure of puberty to occur, short neck, low posterior hairline, narrow maxilla, inner canthal folds, downslanting palpebral fissures, obesity, anomalous auricles, narrow palate, excessive pigmented nevi, blue sclera, iris coloboma, hypotelorism			•			•
13q- additional features include microcephaly, severe cognitive deficiency, short neck, broad nasal root, frontal bossing, hypertelorism, ptosis, colobomata, epicanthal folds, large slanting ears, microphthalmia	•		•	•		

Long Neck

	Speech	Resonance	Voice	Language	Hearing Sensorineural	Hearing Conductive
Proteus Syndrome additional features include enlarged hands and feet, bony projections on skull, large head, multiple hematomas, hyperpigmentation, thickened skin, increased stature, nevi, unilateral or bilateral overgrowth	•	•		•		•

Short Neck

	Speech	Resonance	Voice	Language	Hearing Sensorineural	Hearing Conductive
Albright's Hereditary Osteodystrophy Syndrome additional features include cognitive impairment, cataracts, rounded face, brachydactyly, obesity, small stature, low nasal bridge, delayed dental eruption, enamel hypoplasia, anomalous digits, prognathic profile, vertebral defects, hearing deficit, short limbs, large great toe, small, upturned nose, hypoplastic maxilla	•	•		•		•

	Speech	Resonance	Voice	Language	Hearing Sensorineural	Conductive
Cardio-Facio-Cutaneous Syndrome additional features include large forehead, sparse curly scalp hair, depressed nasal root, ptosis, small stature, hypotonia, cardiac anomalies, posteriorly rotated ears, nystagmus, strabismus, mild-to-moderate mental retardation, shallow orbital ridges, brain anomalies, relative macrocephaly, downslanting palpebral fissures	•	•	•	•		
CHARGE Syndrome additional features include iris coloboma, heart anomalies, choanal atresia, growth retardation, ear anomalies, genital anomalies, nystagmus, micrognathia, cleft lip, facial palsy, mental deficiency	•	•	•	•	•	•
DeLange's Syndrome additional features include short stature, limb reduction, depressed nasal bridge, microcephaly, hypertonia, cleft palate, low anterior hairline, thin upper lip, micrognathia, long curly eyelashes, downturned corners of mouth, high arched palate, mental retardation, bushy eyebrows, hirsutism, clinodactyly of fifth fingers, simian creases, blue sclera, nystagmus, downslanting palpebral fissures	•	•	•	•	•	•
Fetal Hydantoin Syndrome additional features include growth deficiency, cleft palate, cleft lip, short nose, flat philtrum, low anterior hairline, hypoplastic distal phalanges, hirsutism, wide anterior fontanel, ocular hypertelorism, broad nasal bridge, bowed upper lip, cognitive impairment, abnormal palmar crease, coarse hair, low posterior hairline, upslanting palpebral fissures, delayed closure of fontanels	•	•		•		•
Hurler's Syndrome additional features include short stature, dementia, coarse facial features, macroencephaly, corneal clouding, full lips, flared nostrils, low nasal bridge, inner epicanthal folds, retinal pigmentation, cognitive impairment, large tongue, small teeth, joint anomalies, heart anomalies, hirsutism, nystagmus, iris coloboma	•	•	•	•	•	

	Speech	Resonance	Voice	Language	Hearing Sensorineural	Hearing Conductive
Morquio's Syndrome additional features include short stature, corneal clouding, joint and spine anomalies, macrostomia, short nose, widely spaced teeth, coarse facial features, thin enamel on teeth, deep central dimple in chin		•	•		•	•
Noonan's Syndrome additional features include short stature, ptosis of eyelids, low posterior hairline, webbed neck, downslanting eyes, cardiac defect, epicanthal folds, hypertelorism, myopia, nystagmus, strabismus, malocclusion, cognitive impairment, wide mouth, prominent upper lip, retrognathia, low set ears, downslanting palpebral fissures	•	•	•	•	•	•
Opitz's Syndrome additional features include cleft palate, cleft lip, upward or downward slanting palpebral fissures, ocular hypertelorism, broad nasal bridge, cryptorchidism, hypospadias, widow's peak, posterior rotation of auricle, mild-to-moderate mental retardation, hypotelorism	•	•	•	•		•
Scheie's Syndrome additional features include liver enlargement, mild facial coarsening, full lips, broad mouth, deep central dimple in chin, macrostomia, corneal clouding, hirsutism, prognathic mandible, joint limitations			•			•
Trisomy 21/Down's Syndrome additional features include upslanted palpebral fissures, short stature, hypotonia, mental retardation, strabismus, macroglossia, midline parital hair whorl, low posterior hairline, late closure of fontanels, small nose, low nasal bridge, inner epicanthal folds, brushfield spots in iris, hypotelorism, hypertelorism, nystagmus, cardiac anomalies, ear anomalies, protruding ears, microtia	•	•	•	•		•

	Speech	Resonance	Voice	Language	Hearing Sensorineural	Conductive
Turner's Syndrome additional features include short stature, webbed neck, failure of puberty to occur, low posterior hairline, narrow maxilla, inner canthal folds, downslanting palpebral fissures, obesity, anomalous auricles, narrow palate, excessive pigmented nevi, blue sclera, iris coloboma, hypotelorism			•			•
Wildervanck's Syndrome additional features include facial asymmetry, eye motility disorder, nystagmus, epibulbar dermoids, low hairline, preauricular tags and pits	•	•	•	•	•	•
9p- additional features include hypertelorism, cognitive deficiency, microstomia, micrognathia, ear lobe anomalies, craniosynostosis, upslanting palpebral fissures, prominent eyes, higher arched eyebrows, depressed nasal bridge, long philtrum, long middle phalanges of fingers	•	•		•		•
13q- additional features include microcephaly, severe cognitive deficiency, webbed neck, broad nasal root, frontal bossing, hypertelorism, ptosis, colobomata, epicanthal folds, large slanting ears, microphthalmia	•		•	•		
18p- additional features include small stature, microcephaly, hypotelorism, retrognathia, deep central dimple in chin, macrostomia, downturned corners of mouth	•	•		•		

Syndromes With Skin Anomalies
Hyperpigmentation

	Speech	Resonance	Voice	Language	Hearing Sensorineural	Conductive
Berardinelli-Lipodystrophy Syndrome additional features include enlarged liver and heart, cognitive impairment, hirsutism, muscular hypertrophy, tall stature, coarse skin, large superficial veins, absence of facial subcutaneous fat, hypertrophic tonsils and adenoids, curly scalp hair, accelerated growth and maturation, enlarged hands and feet	•	•		•		
Bloom's Syndrome additional features include short stature, cognitive deficiency, psychiatric illness, deficient subcutaneous fat, microcephaly, molar hypoplasia, facial erythema, hypopigmentation, café au lait spots	•		•	•		
Clouston's Syndrome additional features include thickened skin on palms and feet, strabismus, short stature, alopecia, hypoplastic nails, deficient eyelashes and eyebrows	•			•		
Fanconi's Pancytopenia Syndrome additional features include short stature, microcephaly, small or absent thumbs, renal anomalies, strabismus, hypoplastic radii, cognitive impairment, eye anomalies, nystagmus	•			•		•
Proteus Syndrome additional features include enlarged hands and feet, bony projections on skull, large head, multiple hematomas, thickened skin, increased stature, long neck, nevi, unilateral or bilateral overgrowth	•	•		•		•

Hypopigmentation

	Speech	Resonance	Voice	Language	Hearing Sensorineural	Conductive
Bloom's Syndrome additional features include short stature, cognitive deficiency, psychiatric illness, deficient subcutaneous fat, microcephaly, molar hypoplasia, facial erythema, hyperpigmentation, café au lait spots	•		•	•		

	Speech	Resonance	Voice	Language	Hearing Sensorineural	Conductive
Hypohidrotic Ectodermal Dysplasia Syndrome additional features include thin fair skin, alopecia, sparse fine hair, silver hair, hypodontia, small nose, thin and wrinkled eyelids, hypoplastic sweat glands, conical anterior teeth, full forehead, low nasal bridge, full lips	•		•			
Piebaldness additional features include white forelock of hair, hyperpigmented borders between pigmented and unpigmented zones	•	•			•	
Waardenburg Syndrome, Type I additional features include heterochromia, partial albinism, pigmentary anomalies of hair, white forelock, broad and high nasal bridge, broad mandible, full lips, medial flare of eyebrows, short palpebral fissures					•	

Café au Lait Spots

	Speech	Resonance	Voice	Language	Sensorineural	Conductive
Bloom's Syndrome additional features include short stature, cognitive deficiency, psychiatric illness, deficient subcutaneous fat, microcephaly, molar hypoplasia, facial erythema, hypopigmentation, hyperpigmentation	•		•	•		
Louis-Bar's Syndrome additional features include athetosis, progressive ataxia, progressive cognitive deterioration, nystagmus, small stature, telangiectasia over bridge of nose and auricles	•	•	•	•		
Neurofibromatosis-Type I additional features include cutaneous neurofibromas, skeletal anomalies, pigmented iris, heterochromia	•	•	•	•		
Neurofibromatosis-Type II additional features include bilateral acoustic neuromas, CNS tumors, pigmented iris, short stature, cutaneous neurofibromas, heterochromia	•				•	
Neurofibromatosis-Type III additional features include CNS tumors, acoustic neuromas, macroencephaly, optic glioma, short stature, heterochromia	•			•	•	

	Speech	Resonance	Voice	Language	Hearing Sensorineural	Conductive
Russell-Silver Syndrome additional features include small stature, body asymmetry, large cranium with small triangular face, downturned corners of mouth, late closure of anterior fontanel, micrognathia, hyperhidrosis, hypoglycemia, blue sclera, café au lait spots			•			

Nevi

	Speech	Resonance	Voice	Language	Hearing Sensorineural	Conductive
Basal-Cell Nevus Syndrome additional features include macrocephaly, scoliosis, strabismus, basal cell carcinomas, frontoparietal bossing, broad nasal bridge, prognathism, occasional cognitive impairment, sloping narrow shoulders, vertebral anomalies, heavy fused eyebrows, misshapen carious teeth, epidermal cysts, nystagmus	•	•		•		
Proteus Syndrome additional features include enlarged hands and feet, bony projections on skull, large head, multiple hematomas, hyperpigmentation, thickened skin, increased stature, long neck, unilateral or bilateral overgrowth	•	•		•		•
Sturge-Weber Syndrome additional features include seizures, cognitive impairment, cutaneous hemangioma, (usually in a trigeminal facial distribution), limb enlargement, malocclusion	•	•	•	•		
Turner's Syndrome additional features include short stature, webbed neck, failure of puberty to occur, short neck, low posterior hairline, narrow maxilla, inner canthal folds, downslanting palpebral fissures, obesity, anomalous auricles, narrow palate, blue sclera, iris coloboma, hypotelorism			•			•

Syndromes with Skull Anomalies
Craniosynostosis

	Speech	Resonance	Voice	Language	Hearing Sensorineural	Hearing Conductive
Antley-Bixler Syndrome additional features include digital anomalies, kidney anomalies, heart anomalies, proptosis, frontal bossing, dysplastic ears, depressed nasal bridge, brachycephaly, large anterior fontanel, radio-humeral synostosis, femoral bowing, midface hypoplasia, stenotic external auditory canals, finger and joint anomalies, delayed closure of fontanels	•	•		•		•
Apert's Syndrome additional features include syndactyly, hydrocephalus, cognitive impairment, hypertelorism, high forehead, large fontanels with late closure, strabismus, small nose, narrow palate with median groove, downslanting palpebral fissures, occasional cleft palate, irregular fusion of cervical vertebrae, flat facies, shallow orbits, nystagmus, short anterio-posterior craniofacial diameter	•	•	•	•		•
Carpenter's Syndrome additional features include hypertelorism, polydactyly, cognitive impairment, heart anomalies, lateral displacement of inner canthi, inner canthal folds, small stature, flat nasal bridge, optic atrophy, obesity, variable synostosis, brachydactyly of hands, low set malformed ears, high arched palate, large fontanels	•	•		•		
Crouzon's Syndrome additional features include macrocephaly, maxillary hypoplasia, hypertelorism, frontal bossing, upslanting palpebral fissures, low set ears, hypoplastic maxilla, ocular proptosis, nystagmus, mental retardation, iris coloboma, strabismus, optic atrophy, inverted V shape to palate	•	•				•
Saethre-Chotzen Syndrome additional features include acrocephaly, syndactyly of hands and feet, brachycephaly, high forehead, maxillary hypoplasia, deviated nasal septum, hypertelorism, small ears, ptosis of eyelid, large fontanels with delayed closure						•

	Speech	Resonance	Voice	Language	Hearing Sensorineural	Conductive
9p- additional features include hypertelorism, cognitive deficiency, microstomia, micrognathia, ear lobe anomalies, short neck, upslanting palpebral fissures, prominent eyes, higher arched eyebrows, depressed nasal bridge, long philtrum, long middle phalanges of fingers	•	•		•		•

Large Fontanels

	Speech	Resonance	Voice	Language	Hearing Sensorineural	Conductive
Angelman's Syndrome additional features include microcephaly, ataxic arm movements, seizures, cognitive impairment, decreased pigmentation of iris and choroid, maxillary hypoplasia, widely spaced teeth, blond hair, pale blue eyes, optic atrophy, macrostomia, prognathic mandible, inappropriate laughter, absent speech, macrostomia	•					
Apert's Syndrome additional features include syndactyly, hydrocephalus, cognitive impairment, hypertelorism, high forehead, large fontanels with late closure, strabismus, small nose, narrow palate with median groove, downslanting palpebral fissures, occasional cleft palate, irregular fusion of cervical vertebrae, flat facies, shallow orbits, nystagmus, short anterio-posterior craniofacial diameter	•	•	•	•		•
Beckwith-Wiedemann Syndrome additional features include large size at birth, hypotonia, accelerated growth, macroglossia, creases in ear lobes, large ears, preauricular tags and pits, enlarged liver, enlarged spleen, enlarged kidneys, prominent eyes, malocclusion, prognathic mandible, macrosomia, capillary nevus flammeus	•	•	•	•		•
Carpenter's Syndrome additional features include hypertelorism, polydactyly, cognitive impairment, heart anomalies, lateral displacement of inner canthi, inner canthal folds, craniosynostosis, small stature, flat nasal bridge, optic atrophy, obesity, variable synostosis, brachydactyly of hands, low set malformed ears, high arched palate	•	•		•		

	Speech	Resonance	Voice	Language	Hearing Sensorineural	Conductive
Oto-Palato-Digital Syndrome, Type I additional features include hypertelorism, downslanting eyes, small stature, cleft soft palate, micrognathia, microstomia, frontal prominence, delayed closure of fontanels, low set ears, steep naso-basal angulation, small nose, cognitive impairment, hypoplastic facial bones, broad distal phalanges, downslanting palpebral fissures, upslanting palpebral fissures	•	•	•	•		•
Pyknodysostosis additional features include short stature, micrognathia, abnormal teeth, osteosclerosis, delayed closure of sutures, delayed closure of fontanels, prominent nose, narrow grooved palate, delayed eruption of teeth			•	•		
Weaver's Syndrome additional features include thin hair, accelerated growth, skeletal anomalies, macrocephaly, macrostomia, ocular hypertelorism, developmental delay, large protruding ears, camptodactyly, foot deformities, epicanthal folds, long philtrum, broad forehead, downslanting palpebral fissures, coarse and low-pitched voice, progressive spasticity, strabismus	•		•	•		

Delayed Closure of Fontanels

	Speech	Resonance	Voice	Language	Hearing Sensorineural	Conductive
Antley-Bixler Syndrome additional features include digital anomalies, kidney anomalies, heart anomalies, proptosis, frontal bossing, dysplastic ears, depressed nasal bridge, craniosynostosis, brachycephaly, large anterior fontanel, radio-humeral synostosis, femoral bowing, midface hypoplasia, stenotic external auditory canals, finger and joint anomalies	•	•		•		•
Apert's Syndrome additional features include syndactyly, hydrocephalus, cognitive impairment, hypertelorism, high forehead, large fontanels, strabismus, small nose, narrow palate with median groove, downslanting palpebral fissures, occasional cleft palate, irregular craniosynostosis, fusion of cervical vertebrae, flat facies, shallow orbits, nystagmus, short anterio-posterior craniofacial diameter	•	•	•	•		•

	Speech	Resonance	Voice	Language	Hearing Sensorineural	Conductive
Fetal Hydantoin Syndrome additional features include growth deficiency, cleft palate, cleft lip, short nose, flat philtrum, low anterior hairline, hypoplastic distal phalanges, hirsutism, wide anterior fontanel, ocular hypertelorism, broad nasal bridge, bowed upper lip, cognitive impairment, short neck, abnormal palmar crease, coarse hair, low posterior hairline, upslanting palpebral fissures	•	•		•		•
Hallermann-Streiff Syndrome additional features include short stature, micrognathia, small face, thin small pointed nose, nystagmus, sparse scalp hair and eyelashes, frontal and parietal bossing, cataracts, hypoplastic teeth, microphthalmia, blue sclera, alopecia, hypotelorism, iris coloboma, microstomia, downslanting palpebral fissures	•	•	•			
Osteogenesis Imperfecta Type 1 additional features include bone fragility, blue sclera, small face, small stature, late eruption and irregularly placed teeth, thin skin, otosclerosis, blue gray coloration of teeth, postnatal growth deficiency, triangular facial appearance			•		•	•
Oto-Palato-Digital Syndrome, Type 1 additional features include hypertelorism, downslanting eyes, small stature, cleft soft palate, micrognathia, microstomia, frontal prominence, large fontanels low set ears, steep naso-basal angulation, small nose, cognitive impairment, hypoplastic facial bones, broad distal phalanges, downslanting palpebral fissures, upslanting palpebral fissures	•	•	•	•		•
Pyknodysostosis additional features include short stature, micrognathia, abnormal teeth, osteosclerosis, delayed closure of sutures, large fontanels, prominent nose, narrow grooved palate, delayed eruption of teeth			•	•		

	Speech	Resonance	Voice	Language	Hearing Sensorineural	Conductive
Robinow's Syndrome additional features include hypertelorism, macrocephaly, cleft palate, brachydactyly, vertebral and skeletal anomalies, short forearms, short stature, prominent eyes, small upturned nose, large anterior fontanel, long philtrum, downslanting palpebral fissures, triangular mouth with downturned angles, micrognathia, crowded teeth, posteriorly rotated ears, alopecia, microstomia	•	•				•
Russell-Silver Syndrome additional features include small stature, body asymmetry, large cranium with small triangular face, downturned corners of mouth, late closure of anterior fontanel, micrognathia, hyperhidrosis, hypoglycemia, blue sclera, café au lait spots			•			
Saethre-Chotzen Syndrome additional features include acrocephaly, syndactyly of hands and feet, brachycephaly, high forehead, maxillary hypoplasia, deviated nasal septum, hypertelorism, small ears, ptosis of eyelid, craniosynostosis, large fontanels						•
Trisomy 21/Down's Syndrome additional features include upslanted palpebral fissures, short stature, hypotonia, mental retardation, strabismus, short neck, macroglossia, midline parital hair whorl, low posterior hairline, small nose, low nasal bridge, inner epicanthal folds, brushfield spots in iris, hypotelorism, hypertelorism, nystagmus, cardiac anomalies, ear anomalies, protruding ears, microtia	•	•	•	•		•

INDEX